LANCASTER
A Pictorial History

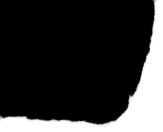
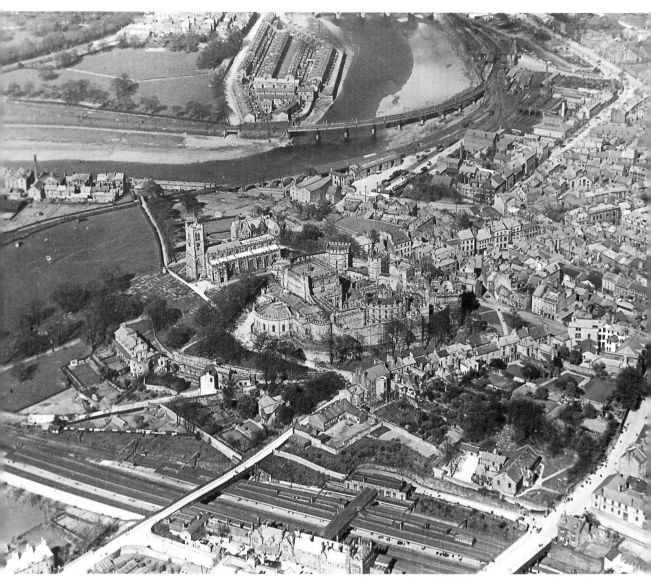

Aerial view of Lancaster from the south-west, taken in the late 1920s. In the foreground is the Castle Station and in the centre the castle and Priory Church. Just visible at the top right hand corner of the picture are Green Ayre Station and Greyhound Bridge which carried the railway line to Morecambe. Greyhound Bridge was converted in about 1973 to carry road traffic.

LANCASTER
A Pictorial History

Andrew White

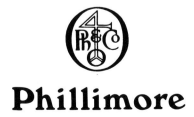

Phillimore

1990

Published by
PHILLIMORE & CO. LTD.
Shopwyke Hall, Chichester, Sussex

ISBN 0 85033 744 5

04581200

Printed and bound in Great Britain by
BIDDLES LTD.
Guildford, Surrey

List of Illustrations

Frontispiece: Aerial view of Lancaster from the south-west in the 1920s

Acknowledgements

All but one of the photographs and other illustrations are drawn from the collections of Lancaster City Museums. Many of the prints are the work of Mr. Albert Gilham, formerly lecturer in photography at Lancaster College of Art. No. 61 is reproduced courtesy of Media Services, University of Lancaster. I should also like to acknowledge the help of my colleagues, Katrina Hunter and Helen Griffiths, in making sense of my manuscript and typing it.

Preface

Despite having lived in Yorkshire, Devonshire and Lincolnshire, I find that I keep returning to Lancaster. My earliest recollections of it are as a child in the early 1950s, being brought here to visit the dentist. Notwithstanding the painful associations, I have always found Lancaster a charming place in which to live and work – small enough to get to know most people, and surrounded by beautiful countryside. I have got to know it especially well during my seven years as Curator of the City's Museums.

A book of this kind is a very personal selection. For every illustration which has gone in there are four or five, equally good, which have had to be left out. A picture book is also very selective from a chronological point of view. Most photographs of Lancaster date from after 1860. Of course, the last 130 years have seen huge changes, and these photographs are of great interest, but our view of the past remains heavily dependent on photographic images. Engravings and maps have been used to take the picture a stage further back, but the fact remains that less than a quarter of Lancaster's 2,000-year history can be shown pictorially.

The main purpose of the book is to introduce new readers to the considerable charm of Lancaster, while providing some unusual views and information for those who already know the area.

Introduction

Lancaster lies at the extreme north of the county that takes its name and, unlike much of that county, has never been overwhelmed by industry. Today it is a pleasant town, set in a beautiful landscape, with Morecambe Bay as its backdrop and the outliers of Bowland Forest rising to the east. In the last century a group of small fishing villages nearby coalesced to form the seaside resort of Morecambe, to the west of Lancaster, while at the same period iron furnaces and the railways created Carnforth, to the north. Lancaster stands on the tidal estuary of the River Lune at its lowest bridging point. To the north-east of the city the Lune valley is a green and peaceful land, with grey stone villages and ancient churches opening on to bare brown fells. The green fields support sheep and dairy cattle.

To understand Lancaster we have to step back 19 centuries in time to the period when it lay at the frontier of the Roman Empire. The advancing Roman army recognised the advantages of the prominent hilltop near a bend in the river where a bridge could be built. Access from the sea meant that the Roman navy could use the Lune to replenish the army's stores, and a fort stood at this strategic position for over three centuries.

On the eastern and northern slopes of the hill, below the fort, a small town grew up. Long, narrow timber buildings housed the wives and children of soldiers, shops, eating houses, and everything the off-duty troops needed. One street in particular, leading from the east gate of the fort, was to be a strong influence on the plan of later Lancaster. It became Church Street, and still forms one of the main thoroughfares. Finds of Roman material throughout the city centre suggest quite a large settlement. Interestingly, no Roman finds have been made in the area of Market Street. Perhaps this was a medieval addition. An excavated Roman bath-house and part of the fort wall can still be seen in Vicarage Field.

> And hard by it standeth upon the height of the hill, the onely Church they have ... a little beneath which, by a faire bridge over Lone, in the descent and side of the hill where it is steepest, hangeth a peece of a most ancient wall of Romane work ...
>
> John Camden, 1610

During the early years of the fifth century the stone fort on the hilltop fell into decay. It no longer served any defensive purpose, but its outer wall survived because of its sheer strength and thickness. The straight lines and regular layout of the Roman houses degenerated into a huddle of smoky huts. Some Roman buildings may have survived, however, their tiled roofs replaced with thatch and their walls patched and mended. Within the ruins of the fort stood the hall of the local chieftain, later to be joined by a primitive church or monastery. Of this the only traces are a handful of *stycas*, the small bronze coins of the period, and carved stone crosses, some of which were built into the later church. The language spoken changed from Latin to Celtic, Old English to Old

Norse; and then new voices were heard, those of the Norman French overlords, who established an earthwork castle within the old Roman fort and rebuilt the church. In 1094 the church became a priory, an English daughter house of the monastery of St Martin, at Seez in Normandy.

Throughout the Middle Ages Lancaster was never more than a small market town. However, not only was it the county town of Lancashire, but it was for many centuries the home of the Assizes. At first these were relatively quiet affairs, but during the Industrial Revolution the population of Lancashire grew until it was one of the densest in Western Europe, with a corresponding increase in crime. The Assizes were also a social occasion, when the gentry came to town and entertained their friends. They took place twice a year, in spring and autumn.

Lancaster Castle was of immense strategic significance but, strangely, it was called to withstand very few sieges. Originally held by Roger de Poitou, the castle became royal property under King John, who rebuilt it in stone, and again in the 14th century. Henry IV was Duke of Lancaster before becoming king, and ever since 1399 the reigning monarch has been heir to the Duchy of Lancaster and the castle has been duchy property.

The town was a border area in the early Middle Ages and belonged to Scotland for a period in the mid-12th century. In 1322 a Scottish raiding army came south and occupied the town for several days, inflicting much damage. A further raid occurred in 1389. The effect was severely to disrupt the economic base of the town and to slow its development.

By the 1260s the Black Friars, or Dominicans, had arrived in Lancaster. Their Friary lay among orchards and gardens to the east of the town. A precinct wall surrounding their property proved a valuable investment when the Scots came in 1322, for the Friary alone, with the Priory, escaped damage. The position of the Friary was to affect the growth of Lancaster. Even after the Dissolution its site blocked eastward expansion and caused the town eventually to grow in upon itself.

By the early 13th century most of the central streets were already in existence, and by the 15th century the process was complete. That is not to say that all the streets were built up. Indeed, many of them would seem very rural and undeveloped to today's residents: citizens had valuable grazing rights on the moors and marshes around, and many kept livestock there.

The 15th century was a time of general decline in English towns. It is hard to tell whether Lancaster shared in this – the records simply do not survive. In the early years of the century the great gatehouse of the castle, one of the best known features of Lancaster, was rebuilt. It bears carved shields with the arms of Henry IV and his son, Henry V. Trade in the town seems to have stagnated for over two and a half centuries, until the wealth of the New World gave it fresh impetus.

The Priory, originally the property of a French monastery, was taken under English control from the end of the 14th century, because of the wars with France. It was given to the nuns of Syon, Middlesex, who wanted little to do with this distant property other than to collect rents. The Priory, from 1430 a parish church with a vicar and a new tithe barn, was rebuilt in the perpendicular style, removing most of the traces of the earlier monastic buildings. One of Lancaster's most prominent citizens at this time was John Gardyner. He took over the lease of Syon's Mill at Newton, one mile up river from Lancaster, and devoted its proceeds to the founding of a Free Grammar School in the churchyard, and to the establishment of a chantry in the parish church, with almshouses for four poor men. Gardyner's estate, at Bailrigg, three miles south of Lancaster, was five centuries later to become the site of Lancaster University.

In 1562 the Chancellor of the Duchy of Lancaster examined the state of the castle. A drawing of the castle and Priory Church, one of the fruits of his work, survives in the Public Record Office. It is the earliest drawing to show the town. Twenty years later the threat from Spain led to the raising and strengthening of the Lungess Tower, the old Norman keep of the castle. The date 1585 and RA, the initials of Ralph Assheton who was responsible for the work, can still be seen below the battlements on the north side.

The earliest plan of the town, by John Speed, was made in 1610. It is not very good, but its early date gives it considerable interest. It shows a layout which is still completely recognisable today, but with gardens and open spaces between the streets which have long been built over. It is likely that the map of 1610 largely reflects the late medieval street plan. Street names have changed in some cases – Kemps Lane and Kelne Lane appear where now we have King Street and China Street – but other names are still familiar. One of these streets, Penny Street, was to see severe damage during the Civil War. In 1643 the Earl of Derby brought a Royalist army against Lancaster Castle. Finding his way blocked by improvised barricades, he burnt down a number of timber buildings in Penny Street. The castle fell to him, but the triumph was short-lived. Lancaster and other Royalist strongholds in the Lune Valley, Hornby and Thurland Castles, were overcome by Parliamentary troops in the following year.

... we entered into the famous county Palatine of Lancaster, by a fayre, lofty, long Archt Bridge, over the River Lun, wee were for the George in Lancaster ...   Captain William Howard, 1634

The deliberate burning of Penny Street in 1643 was matched by the accidental burning of Church Street in 1690. The largely timber-framed buildings fell an easy victim to the flames, and a long list of householders petitioned for relief – there was at that time no fire insurance. One of the effects of this was the gradual rebuilding of Lancaster in stone. Substantial houses with stone party walls made their appearance, and many still survive, even if their façades have been modernised since. William Stout, a prominent Quaker merchant, was to complain in 1739 that he could not find a builder because they were in such demand. The rebuilding was largely paid for by the profits of a new trade. In the 1670s a handful of Lancaster merchants awoke to the fact that they were extremely well placed for trade with the American colonies and with the West Indies. Private quays were built by various merchants on a formerly vacant area of land in the bend of the river above the bridge, known as the Green Ayre. By the 1750s a Port Commission had been established and a new quay, known as St George's Quay, began operations.

The situation of Lancaster town is very good, the Church neately built of stone, the Castle which is just by, both on a very great ascent from the rest of the town and so is in open view ... Lancaster town is old and much decay'd.   Celia Fiennes, 1698

The next 50 years were a time of great prosperity for Lancaster. The wealth of the West Indies poured into the coffers of the merchant families and trade was stimulated all round. As well as ship-building by firms such as Brockbanks and Smiths, there was sailcloth weaving, sail making, rope making and anchor smithing. The town was virtually self-sufficient for such things. Ships of up to 550 tons were built on the river, while those of 200-300 tons regularly came up to the quays to unload sugar, tobacco, rum, coffee, spices, timber and dye-stuffs which were imported and then processed in the port. The family firm of Gillow made fine furniture, much of it from imported mahogany which was in some cases re-exported to adorn the houses of wealthy plantation owners in the West Indies.

You will be pleased with your approach to Lancaster. Ships of 300 tons burthen are navigable up the Lun, about seven miles, to that town. A complete quay wall of 200 yards length, with wharfs, built within these seven years ... The Castle, which is pretty intire, is their county gaol. A delightful prospect from the Church Yard which is on the same hill.   John Crofts, 1759

This wealth had its outward manifestation in the fine stone houses and public buildings which are still a feature of Lancaster. During the course of the 18th century much of the town was rebuilt, so that traces of earlier buildings have disappeared or survive only at the backs or in the roof-structures of outwardly Georgian houses. Stone masons flourished at this time. Much of the stone came from Lancaster Moor, where many of the masons leased stone-quarries from the Corporation. Many streets are still almost wholly Georgian in appearance, especially those around the castle. The castle itself was extensively rebuilt at this time, and was used as a prison. Lancashire, formerly one of the most thinly populated counties in the country, grew immensely as a result of the Industrial Revolution. Its crime rate also went up and, as the seat of the Assizes, Lancaster was where the guilty – and sometimes the innocent – were tried and met their deaths. At Assize time the gentry came to town and entertained their friends. For this purpose many had houses specially built. Ground floors were used for entertainment, the living accommodation being at first-floor level. An Assembly Room was built in King Street.

Communications were improved by the turnpike trusts such as the Garstang to Heron Syke and the Lancaster to Richmond turnpikes, while the advent of the Lancaster Canal in 1797, largely as a result of the money and enthusiasm of Lancaster merchants, still further benefited the distribution of goods made in and traded through the town.

The new houses are peculiarly neat and handsome, the streets are well paved, and thronged with inhabitants, busied in a prosperous trade to the West Indies, and other places. Along a fine quay noble ware-houses are built.   Thomas West, 1793

Prosperity came to an end fairly abruptly as a result of two factors: the ruinous wars with France, which by 1800 had caused a slump in Lancaster's shipping trade, and the failure of the two local banks in the 1820s, which took with them some £420,000 of local savings. Lancaster merchants took their shipping to Liverpool and elsewhere. Farmers felt the pinch of an agricultural decline in the 1820s and 1830s, and many emigrated to the U.S.A. and Canada.

One of the last areas of the town to be developed before the slump was Dalton Square and adjoining streets on what had been the Frierage Estate. Progress was slow; although the development began in 1784, it was far from complete by 1824 when the impetus ran out. Indeed, there are still many gaps and inferior buildings in what was to have been the first of a series of London-type squares.

Another easy stage brought us to Lancaster, one of the best built cities in the Kingdom. The view as we left it after dinner was truly fine; two stone bridges over the river Lon, the town on the opposite bank, and on the highest part of the hill a castle, which has been newly built or repaired as a prison – Lancaster could scarcely have appeared more beautiful in the days of the shield and the lance.
                                             Robert Southey, 1807

Between 1802 and 1864 a number of mills made their appearance, mainly to the south and east of the town. Cotton spinning was the principal activity, but Lancaster was never as dependent upon the textile trade as other Lancashire towns.

Apart from the gradual infill of the older streets, the next 30 years produced little visible change in Lancaster. In 1840 the Lancaster and Preston Junction Railway arrived, with its terminus in South Road (known then as Penny Street Station). The modest station building survives as the nurses' home for the Royal Lancaster Infirmary. It had a short life, being replaced within six years by a new station, Castle Station, on a loop to the west of the town which allowed trains to run through to Carlisle. The Lune was crossed by a high-level bridge, Carlisle Bridge, which has since been rebuilt twice and still carries all the main west coast rail traffic.

Mr Goodchild concludes Lancaster to be a pleasant place, a place dropped in the middle of a charming landscape, a place with a fine ancient fragment of a castle, a place of lively walks, a place possessing staid old houses richly fitted with old Honduras mahogany, which has grown so dark with time that it seems to have got something of a retrospective mirror quality into itself, and to show the visitor, in the depth of its grain, through all its polish, the hue of the wretched slaves who groaned long ago under old Lancaster merchants.   Charles Dickens, 1857

It is probable that the railway brought some prosperity to Lancaster, though it also carried the prosperity away from the port, which continued to decay by degrees. The building of the 'little' North Western Railway through the Lune Valley led to the growth of a number of works on the riverbank, one of which was the Wagon Works. This vast area of buildings housed a most successful concern which produced wagons for railways all over the world. It was one of a number of new industries developed during the 19th century. Another of these was the Lune Shipbuilding Company, set up to build iron ships down at the New Quay. The wooden shipbuilding trade of Lancaster had long since disappeared. The Lune Shipbuilding Company was not a great success and lasted only seven years, though it was responsible for a number of fine vessels. Its bankruptcy allowed a new entrepreneur to buy land cheap down the river at New Quay and use it as a basis for building new works. This was James Williamson.

James Williamson the elder started the great company which his son, later Lord Ashton, was to develop in a very great way. Williamson Senior had invented in 1844 a table baize 'that could stand wear as well as criticism'. The firm went on to produce not only table baize but floor cloths and linoleum, and linoleum was to be their biggest item of sale. The firm controlled all aspects of its work, firing bricks to build its factory, making its own machinery and importing the raw materials, overseeing every stage of the process. In 1862 the firm gave a Christmas dinner for 70 workers, but by the time of James Williamson Senior's death in 1879 the number employed had risen to 2,000. By 1911, Williamson & Sons employed almost a quarter of Lancaster's working men, as well as many women. Storey Bros. & Co. were in competition with Williamsons and formed in many ways the other half of a very polarised town. By 1909 Storeys were probably employing only half the number of men in the Williamsons' pay. In 1892 the two firms agreed to limit their range of products to avoid unnecessary competition. However, it was not merely as great entrepreneurs that the two families were in competition, but also in politics (Storey was a Conservative, while Williamson was a Liberal) and in the field of public generosity. Lord Ashton gave the Ashton Memorial, Wiliamson Park, the Queen Victoria monument in Dalton Square, and the Town Hall, as well as many other smaller gifts. Storeys, for their part, gave the Storey Institute in Market Street as a School of Art and Art Gallery with a Technical School added later, as well as supporting the hospital and Grammar School.

The coming of the railways also helped to foster the growth of Morecambe. Four miles distant from Lancaster, it had its origin in a group of seaside fishing villages set back a little way from the coast. These were Poulton-le-Sands, Torrisholme and Bare. When the railway arrived at what was then a small watering place, development proceeded swiftly. The change of name to Morecambe, from the bay of the same name, did not take effect until about the 1860s. Morecambe itself as an entity only dates from the end of the century. Fishing took place alongside the more traditional seaside activities. Piers were added in 1872 and 1896, along with other seaside facilities. Much of the original prosperity of Morecambe arose from the catching of Morecambe Bay shrimps which, packed in butter, were served at many a Victorian tea table.

Further down the coast, Heysham was not involved in this first growth and retains some of its village charm, as well as the only two Anglo-Saxon churches in Lancashire. While Morecambe was growing so, too, was Lancaster. The original urban core of a few streets developed inwards and many yards and courts grew up containing small unpretentious buildings occupying what had once been gardens. In the course of time these degenerated and in many cases became insanitary slums. However, the town later began to grow outwards and new areas were developed. One of these was the Freehold, an area where all the property was built on land owned by the Freehold Land Company. Another area to be developed lay along South Road and the Greaves, where the early and mid-19th-century villas of successful Lancaster tradesmen and merchants stood in large gardens, but in due course speculative builders took over. Terraces were built along the main road, now the A6, much of the way to Scotforth. Scotforth itself was still a separate village with its own distinctive atmosphere. Skerton, the suburb north of the river, also had the character of a village.

None of the mill owners, such as Storeys or Williamsons, built any housing for their workers. Most of the workers lived in cheaper houses all over the town. Some of the managers of Williamsons lived in larger houses in the more salubrious suburbs. However, there was as yet a very limited middle class in Lancaster, due to its industrialisation during the 19th century which had drawn in large numbers of unskilled and semi-skilled labourers.

The Dispensary movement of the 18th century, which had seen provision of very basic medical facilities for the poor, developed in the 19th century into a whole series of hospitals. In 1816, for instance, the County Asylum was built on land beyond Lancaster Moor and this was followed by others such as the Royal Albert Asylum and the Ripley Hospital. In 1896 the Royal Lancaster Infirmary was opened, the first modern type of hospital in Lancaster. In 1870s and 1880s the Cardwell army reforms led to the building of Bowerham Barracks. This served as the depot for the 4th Foot or King's Own Royal Lancaster Regiment, and fulfilled this role until 1959. A Militia Barracks had been built in South Road in 1859, and later this became part of Storeys White Cross Mill complex.

The Royal Grammar School, which was founded in the Middle Ages, outgrew its original site in the churchyard and in 1851 was moved to a new site in East Road. In 1964 the University of Lancaster was opened and with it an associated college for teacher training, St Martin's College, in the former Bowerham Barracks. The university has had an immense effect on the economic and cultural life of the area. In the 20th century education and health have been the two principal employers in Lancaster. Increasingly, service industries have taken over from the manufacturing industries of the past, though gas derived from a gas-field below Morecambe Bay and electricity from nuclear power stations at Heysham are an important power source and provide considerable employment.

In 1937 Lancaster was awarded city status, on account of its ancient origins and royal associations. The status is honorary, and does not greatly affect its constitution or finance. In 1974 five former local authorities joined together to form a new Lancaster City Council. This occupies exactly the same area as the ancient Hundred of Lonsdale South of the Sands. Today Lancaster is strategically placed on the transport network, lying as it does on both the M6 motorway and the main west coast railway line. It is entering a new period of prosperity brought about by tourism, and businesses are also being encouraged to relocate here.

*   *   *

The photographs and other illustrations in this book are all drawn from the collections of Lancaster City Museums. Many of the photographs are by Sam Thompson (1871-1945), who recorded the changing face of Lancaster and, in particular, the demolition of the yards and courts in the 1920s and 1930s. The man in a bowler hat, carrying a bag, who appears frequently, is Jim Rowe, Sam Thompson's friend and assistant, who was introduced to give human scale.

Bibliography

Ashworth, S., *The Lino King: The Life and Times of Lord Aston* (Huntington, 1989).

Birtwistle, J. M., *Skerton in Times Past* (Brinscall, 1983).

Brownbill, J., & Nuttall, J. R., *A Calendar of Charters and Records belonging to the Corporation of Lancaster* (Lancaster, 1929).

Champness, J., *A New Walk around Historic Lancaster* (Lancaster, 1986).

Champness, J., *Lancashire's Architectural Heritage* (Preston, 1988).

Clark, C., *An Historical and Descriptive Account of the Town of Lancaster* (Lancaster, 1807).

Collingwood, W. G., *Northumbrian Crosses of the Pre-Norman Age* (London, 1927).

Docton, K., *Lancaster as it Was* (Nelson, 1973).

Janes, D .C., *Old Towns and Cities ... Lancaster* (Clapham, 1974).

Jones, G. D. B., & Shotter, D. C. A. *Roman Lancaster: Rescue Archaeology in An Historic City, 1970-75* (Manchester, 1988).

Lancaster City Council, *The City of Lancaster* (Lancaster, 1987).

Pape, T., *The Charters of the City of Lancaster* (Lancaster, 1952).

Penney, S., *Lancaster: the Evolution of its Townscape to 1800* (University of Lancaster, Occasional Paper No. 9, 1981).

Penney, S., *Lancaster in Old Picture Postcards* (Zaltbommel, 1983).

Price, J. W. A., *The Industrial Archaeology of the Lune Valley* (University of Lancaster, Occasional Paper No. 13, 1983).

Rigbye, R. E. K., 'Cross Fleury', *Time Honoured Lancaster* (Lancaster, 1891).

Roberts, E. A. M., *Working Class Barrow and Lancaster, 1890 to 1930* (University of Lancaster, Occasional Paper No. 2, 1976).

Roper, W. O., *Materials for the History of the Church of Lancaster* (Chetham Soc., Manchester, 4 vols., 1892-1906).

Roper, W. O., *Materials for the History of Lancaster* (Lancaster, 1907).

Shotter, D., & White, A., *Roman Fort and Town of Lancaster* (University of Lancaster, Occasional Paper No. 18, 1990).

Simpson, R., *The History and Antiquities of the Town of Lancaster* (Lancaster, 1852).

Whincop, A., & White, A., *Lancaster's Maritime Heritage* (Lancaster, 1986).

White, A. J. (ed.), *The Beauties of the North: Lancaster in 1820* (Lancaster, 1989).

Setting the Scene

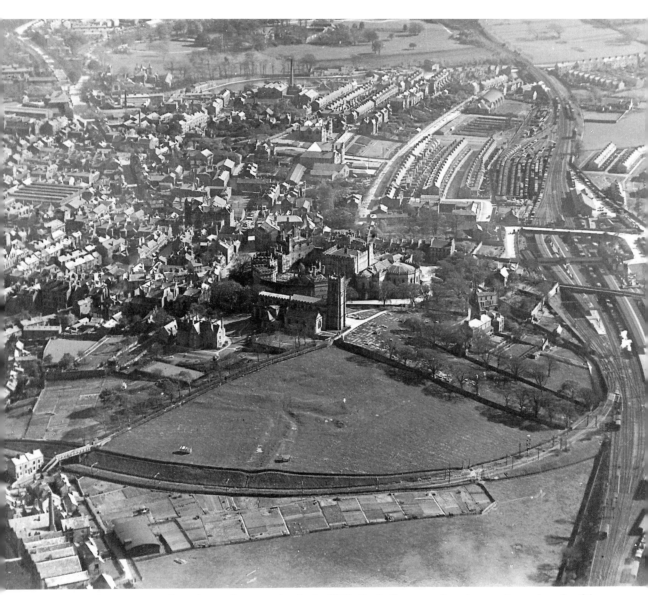

1. Aerial view of Lancaster from the north-west, taken in the 1920s. In the foreground can be seen the earthworks of the Roman fort and the medieval Priory precinct in the Vicarage Fields. The eastern Vicarage Field at this date was still under allotments, below which is the link line between Green Ayre and Castle stations.

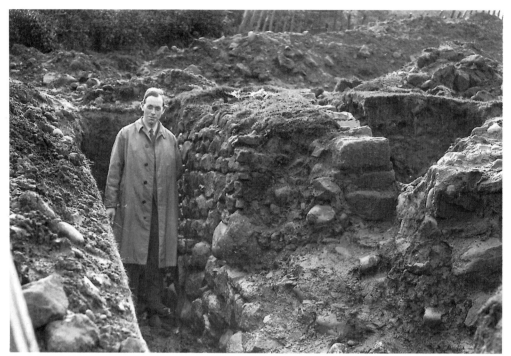

2.   Excavations in progress on the Vicarage Fields between 1927 and 1929. Gilbert Bland, the former Borough Librarian and Curator, is standing in a deep trench beside the walls of a building which was probably part of a medieval gatehouse to Lancaster Priory. The excavations were very extensive but produced few clues as to the layout of the Roman fort.

3.   Excavations nearly completed on the Vicarage Fields, 1973-5. These excavations located a courtyard building whose south wing was a stone-built bath house. A large house, perhaps belonging to a Roman official, is believed to have stood on this site. The bath house element can be seen in the foreground with the remains of its under-floor heating system. It is cut through by a wide and deep V-shaped ditch which dates from the mid-fourth century A.D. and runs alongside the massive Wery Wall which dominated the whole site. The bath house and courtyard building were demolished in the course of building this great defensive wall, belonging to the last fort upon the site. The site has since been consolidated and can still be seen.

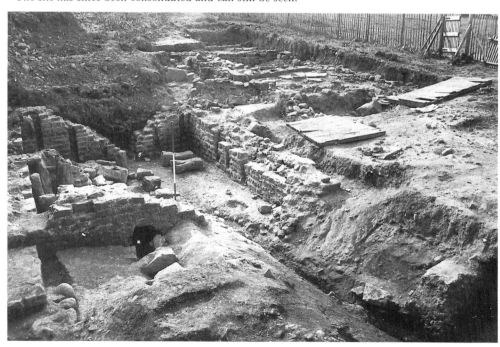

4. Roman pottery vessels found in the Roman civilian settlement outside the fort at Lancaster. These include: rear left, a mortarium for grinding and preparing food; rear right, a burial urn, probably found on the site of St Thomas' church; left front, two beakers; and right front, three flagons for water or wine. All are in Lancaster City Museum.

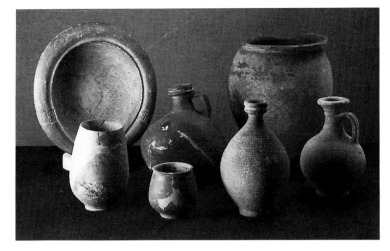

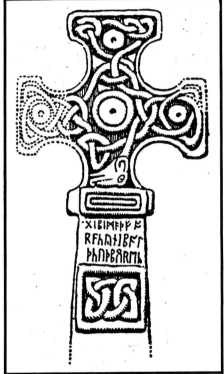

5. Anglian runic cross, found in the Priory churchyard in 1807, and now in the British Museum. The inscription reads 'pray for the soul of Cynibalth, (son of) Cuthber ...'.

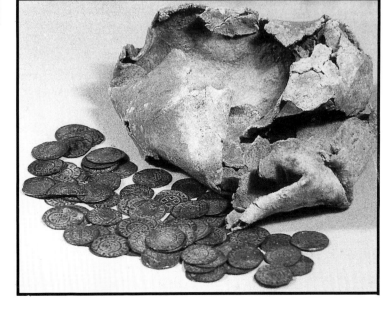

6. Part of a hoard of 86 silver pennies and halfpennies found in a lead wrapper at Scotforth in 1854. The precise findspot is not known, but may have been in the vicinity of Belle View. The coins date from the reigns of Henry II and Richard I, and were probably deposited around A.D. 1196.

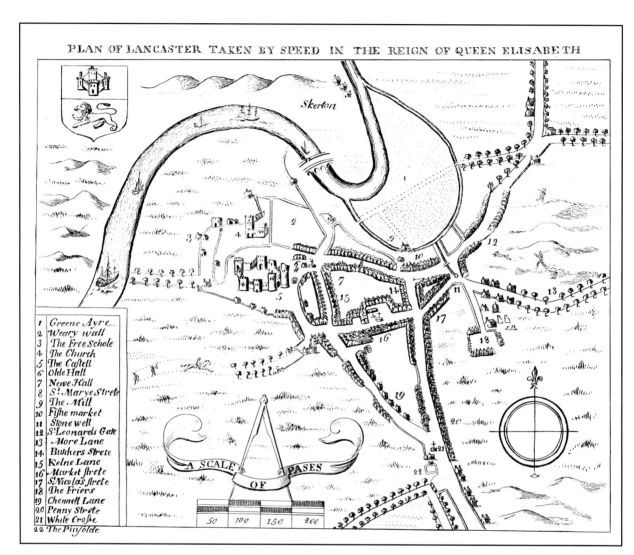

Skerton

1	Greene Ayre
2	Weary wall
3	The Free Schole
4	The Church
5	The Castell
6	Olde Hall
7	Newe Hall
8	St. Marye Strete
9	The Mill
10	Fishe market
11	Stone well
12	St Leonards Gate
13	More Lane
14	Butchers Strete
15	Kelne Lane
16	Market strete
17	St Nicolas Strete
18	The Friers
19	Chennell Lane
20	Penny Strete
21	White Crosse
22	The Pinsolde

A SCALE OF PASES

50   100   150   200

7.   A map of Lancaster in 1610 by John Speed. It shows a very small and open town centre with large gardens behind the houses. It is the earliest surviving map of Lancaster, and probably shows a townscape little different from that of the Middle Ages.

8. The imposing gatehouse of Lancaster Castle, with its portcullis, oak gates and wicket. The shields at the top are of Henry IV and his son, the future Henry V, showing that the gatehouse belongs to the early 15th century. Over the gate is a statue of John O'Gaunt, father of Henry IV, added in 1822. The sculptor was Claud Nimmo.

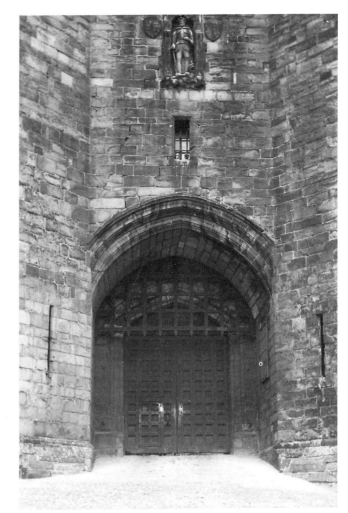

9. From time to time traces of earlier timber buildings are found within more modern stone structures in Lancaster. These cruck frames were found in 1988 when demolition work took place on Mitchell's old brewery in Church Street. The building lay behind the *New Inn* and was probably built in the 17th century.

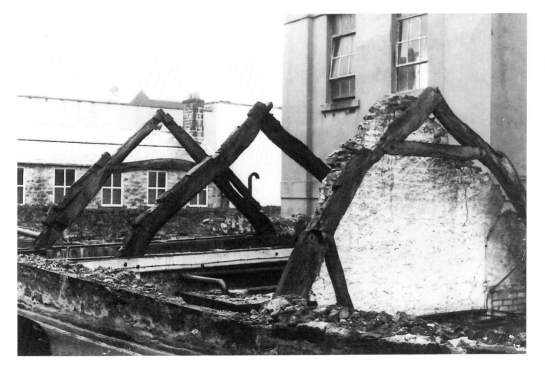

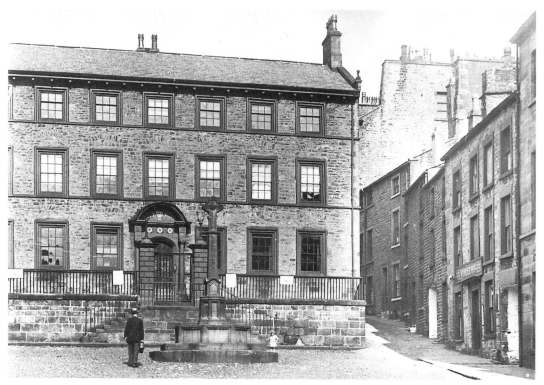

10. The Judges' Lodging, now a museum. Built by Thomas Covell, the governor of Lancaster Castle, this early 17th-century building was very much in advance of its time. The sash windows are later, but many of the roof timbers show the character of the original building. In front of the building is the Covell Cross, re-erected on its medieval site in 1902 in honour of the coronation of Edward VII.

11. Penny's Hospital, built in 1720 under the terms of the will of the late Alderman William Penny. These 12 almshouses and a chapel lie on the west side of King Street and were completely restored in 1974. The Assembly Room next door was built as a place of entertainment and to provide funds for the running of Penny's Hospital. Today the management is in the hands of Lancaster United Charities.

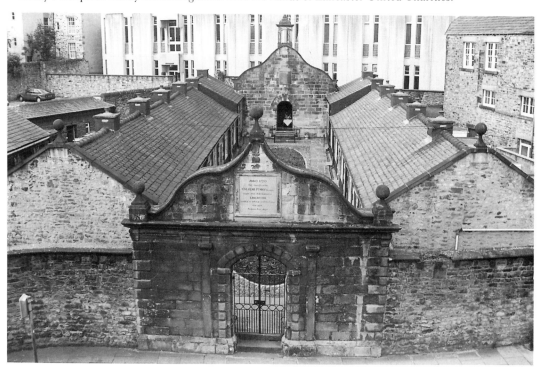

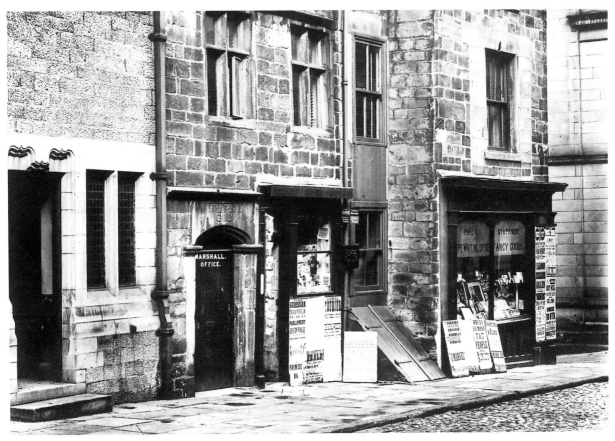

12. Church Street. The building to the left is the masonic hall; that to the right was the house of George Foxcroft, with a door lintel dated 1684. This fine example of vernacular building has been replaced by a modern extension to the masonic hall.

13. The end of China Lane where it emerged into Church Street, in or before 1895. The fine building in the centre of the picture has long gone and is typical of late 17th-century vernacular architecture in Lancaster.

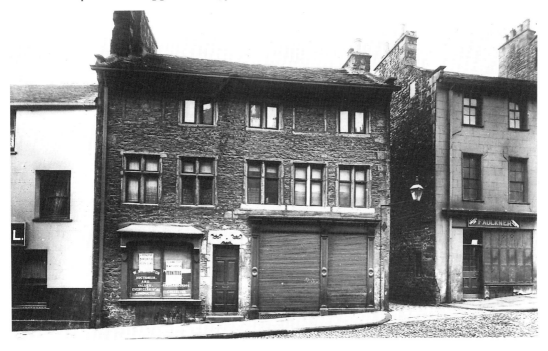

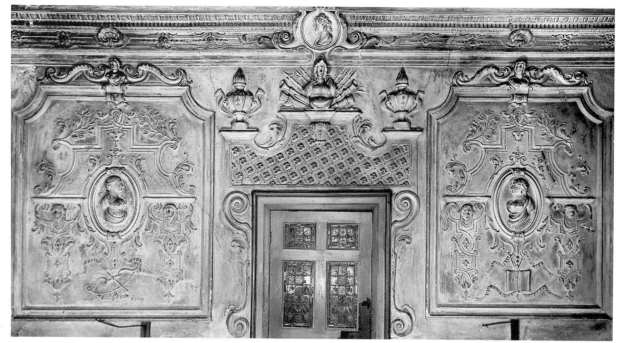

14. Details of the plasterwork in the music room, Sun Street. This superb work, dating from the 1730s, and by Italian craftsmen, is seen here before restoration began in 1974. The building was originally constructed as a summer house of grand proportions, in the garden of Mr. Marton. When the gardens were sold off as building land in 1797, this role was lost. It served for many years as a draughtsmen's office and as a store for heating pipes. It was rescued at the eleventh hour by the Landmark Trust, who restored it to splendid condition and now open it to the public.

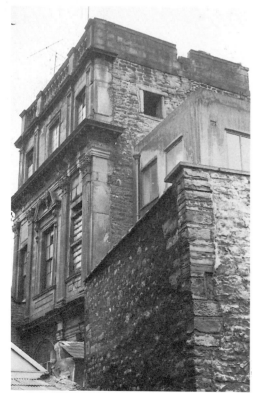

15. The Music Room, in Sun Street, prior to restoration in 1974-5. This magnificent building was long used as a workshop and a mass of unsightly buildings were placed against its front. As well as the restoration work, carried out by the Landmark Trust, Lancaster City Council cleared away the derelict buildings in front and produced a most attractive square, called Sun Street Square.

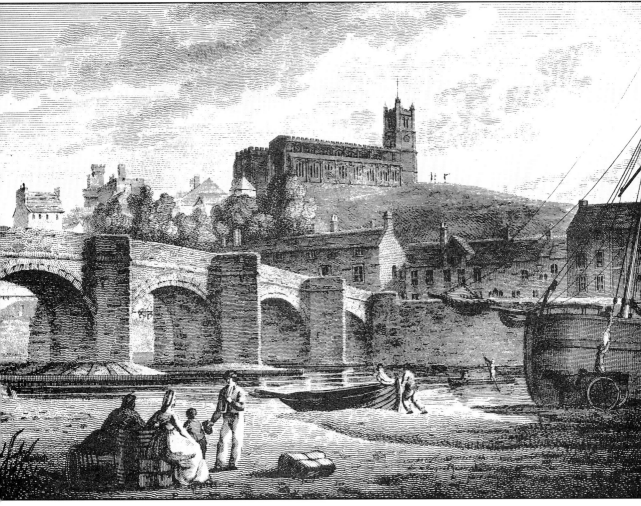

16. Lancaster Old Bridge in 1797, from an engraving by J. Walker after Dayes. The bridge survived until 1802, when its first arch was removed. It was formerly the main access route to the north from Lancaster and all traffic had to pass over it. The building of Skerton Bridge in 1788 rendered it redundant. The last arch fell in 1846 and now there is little or no evidence of it. In the background can be seen the Priory Church on the hilltop, and below it and slightly to the left a little octagonal summer house which stands in the garden of Grey Court, St Marygate.

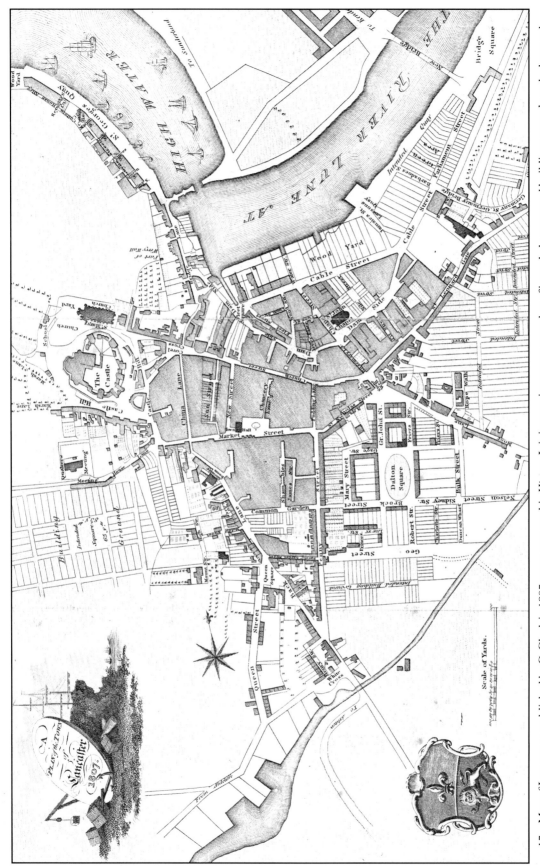

17. Map of Lancaster, published by C. Clark in 1807 to accompany his *History*. It is interesting to see a number of intended streets and building ground marked around the then built up area. Little or nothing of this development took place in the form shown on the map. Nineteenth-century working-class housing occupies these spaces now.

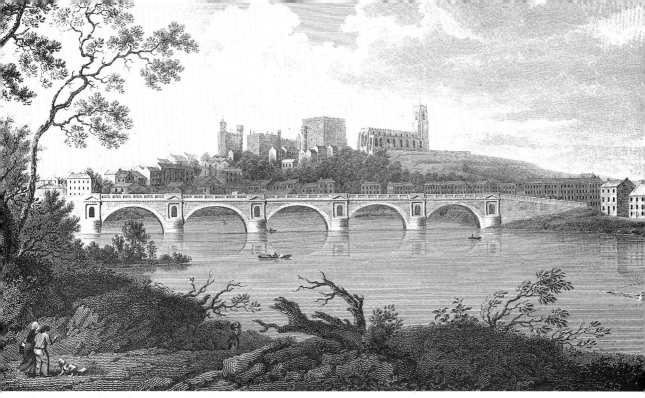

18. Skerton Bridge, the castle and the Priory Church in 1791, engraved by Landseer after J. Farington. Skerton Bridge was very new at this time, and its clean, unblackened lines can be made out very clearly. Farington painted a number of watercolours from this viewpoint.

19. **Lancaster** from Green Ayre, after J. C. Ibbotson, 1807. This view is similar to the 1840s' view, but from further along Cable Street. Brockbank's shipyard appears on the right. A number of Georgian buildings, including No. 1 Water Street (in the centre of the picture), can still be identified. Note the rural appearance of Lancaster at this time, with cattle and pigs in the main street.

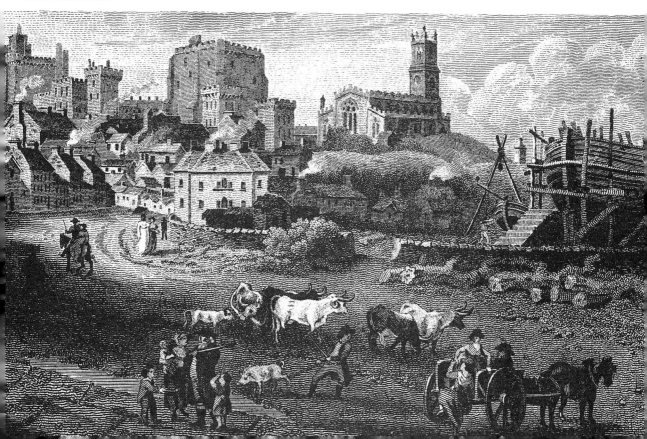

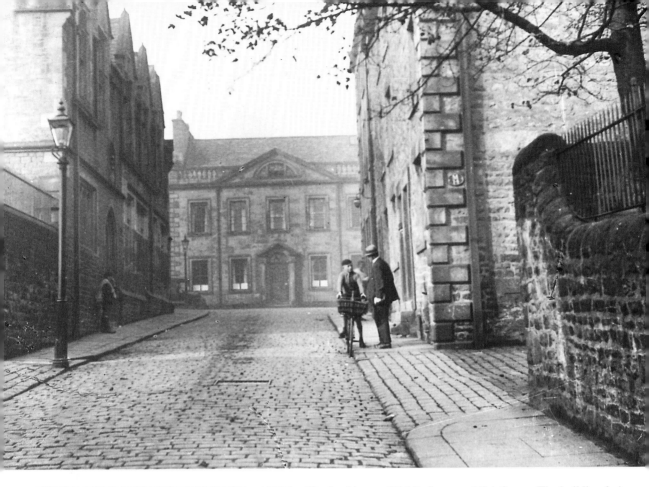

20. Looking up Middle Street to High Street. The building facing down the street is the former St Anne's Vicarage, one of the finest Georgian houses in Lancaster. On the left is the former Girls' Charity School. Lancaster's High Street, unlike that of many towns, is a quiet backwater rather than the main street.

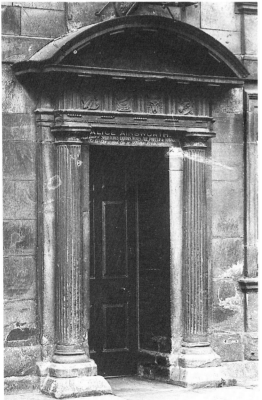

21. The doorway of the *Ring O'Bells Hotel* in King Street. One of the finest Georgian doorways in Lancaster, it has a series of trophies carved over its head. The hotel was probably once a private house.

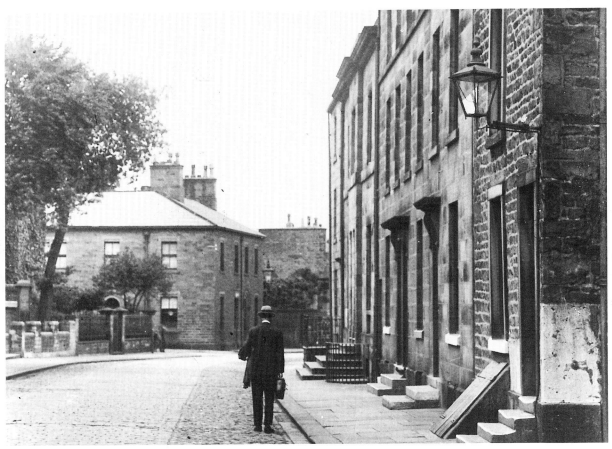

22. Queen Street in 1927. This was one of the areas developed for residential purposes in the Georgian period, and fine houses can be seen on both sides.

23. Queen Square, *c.*1927. The house in the picture is a very dignified building called Falcon House. Queen Square is actually a triangle, not a proper square, leading off King Street. Like many other developments it owes its shape to the pre-existing shape of the fields it replaced.

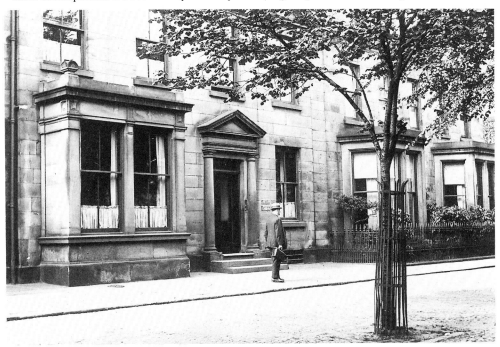

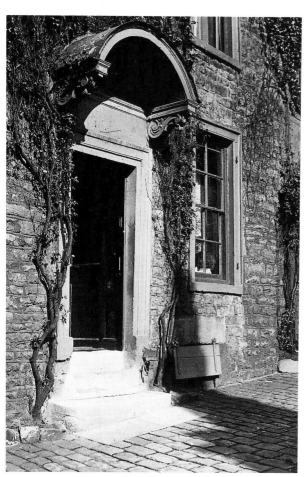

24. The doorway of a house on St Mary's Parade. The artist Reginald Aspinwall lodged here. Until about the 1940s these houses stood on the left, below the Priory Church steps, as a continuation of the surviving St Mary's Parade. They gradually fell into decay and were eventually demolished.

25. Cable Street photographed in 1927. The whole of this area has been influenced by the building of the bus station just before the Second World War. The fine houses on the right hand side were built for merchants and gentry from the 1750s onwards. The railings and steps in the right foreground have now disappeared. The buildings at the centre of the picture, Nos. 1 and 2 Cable Street, were built by Richard Gillow, a well-known cabinet maker. No. 1 was the house of Captain Henry Fell. This building has suffered more recently from the demolition of its upper storeys.

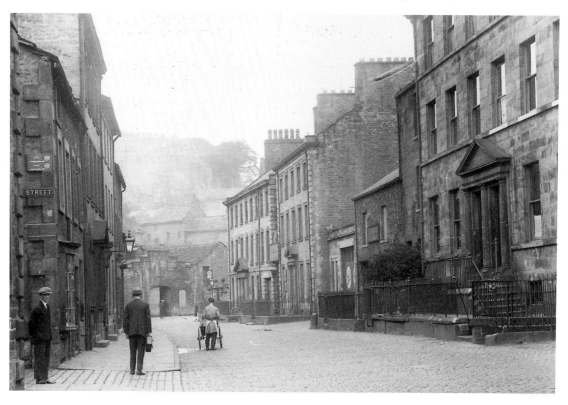

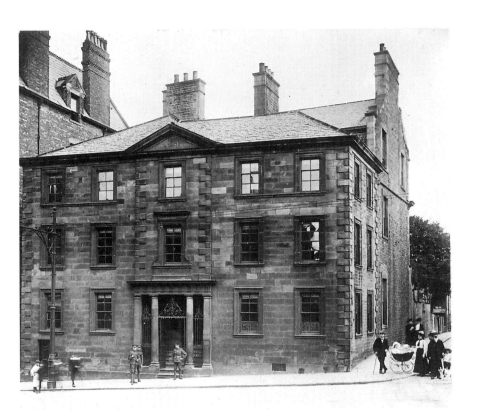

26. The house of Mr. John Fenton-Cawthorne, M.P. for Lancaster, at the junction of Meeting House Lane and Fenton Street. Built in 1806, it was demolished in 1921 to make way for the post office. Parts of the centre bay survive, built into the Storey Institute opposite. Mr. Fenton-Cawthorne's country estate was at Wyreside Hall.

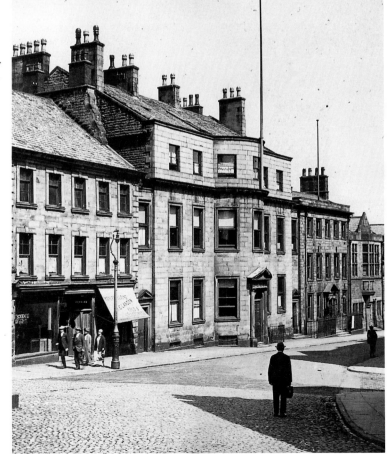

27. Church Street, before the demolition of properties in Bridge Lane in order to realign the road. There are a number of fine buildings in this view, two of which survive. Dr. Daniel Wilson's house (with the bow front) was built in 1772. The present Conservative Club, to its right, was built as a town house of the Marton family in the early 18th century. Church Street was one of the principal streets in the 18th century and many of the gentry had their town houses in this area.

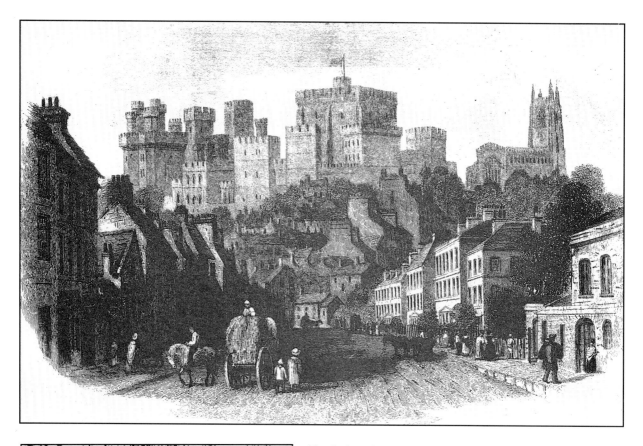

28. A view of Lancaster Castle and Priory Church from Cable Street, *c.*1840. The original steel engraving captures very well, even if it exaggerates, the mass of buildings on the hilltop. The castle has been deliberately increased in scale to render it more impressive.

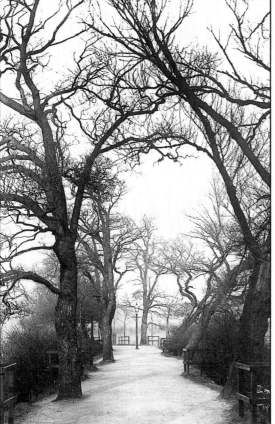

29. Ladies' Walk before the First World War. This pleasant rural walk through an avenue of trees marked the north-eastern edge of Lancaster's built-up area. The 'ladies' of Ladies' Walk are almost certainly the nuns of Syon Abbey in Middlesex, who acquired the Priory Church in the late 14th century and owned property in the area, particularly fishing rights and a mill on the Lune.

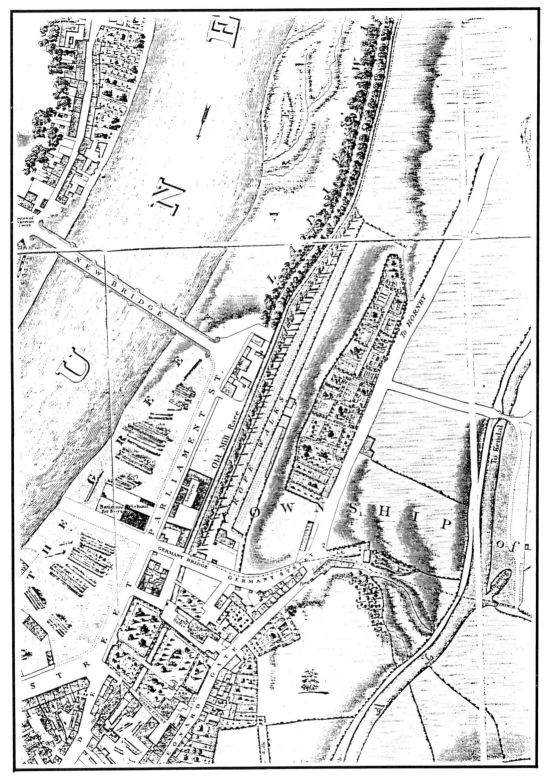

30. Detail from Jonathan Binns' map of Lancaster, 1821, showing the riverside area around Skerton Bridge (the 'new bridge'). The old mill-race shows up very clearly, as does the rope walk, the buildings of which still survive. Beyond the toll house can be seen Ladies' Walk, which disappeared during reconstruction work in the First World War.

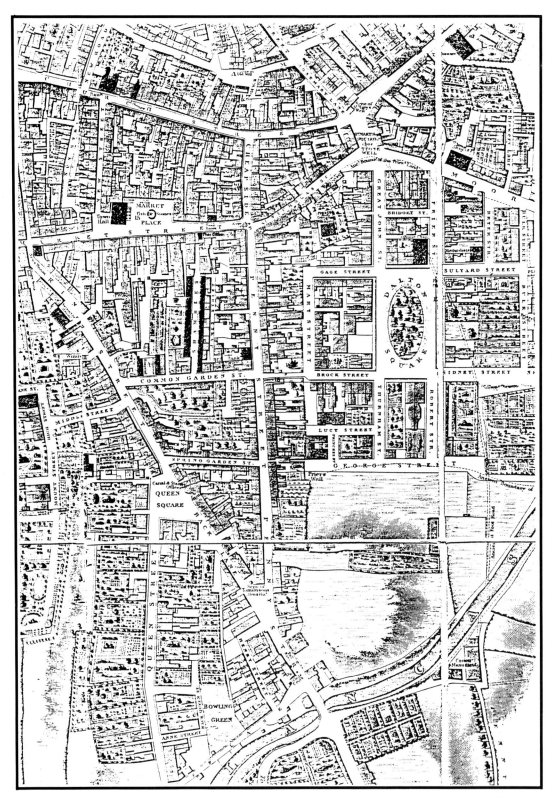

31. Detail of Jonathan Binns' map of Lancaster, 1821, showing the Dalton Square area. By this time Dalton Square was virtually as built up as it is now. Two large houses fronting onto the Square between Robert Street and Thurnham Street were later named Nazareth House and in 1909 this became the site of the new Town Hall. The Methodist church in Sulyard Street marks the site of the former Dominican Friary. The names of the various streets around Dalton Square are taken from members of the Dalton family, who developed the area.

32. A section of Harrison & Hall's map of Lancaster in 1877, showing the Freehold Estate. The road names are all taken from the Lake District and their plots follow a similar, though not uniform, shape. Various gaps can be seen in the building line, where other buildings were later fitted in. Moor Lane and Bath Street were in existence before the Freehold Estate and the building at the end of Bath Street was originally the Cold Bath, built by subscription in 1803. When it was opened it stood on the edge of open countryside.

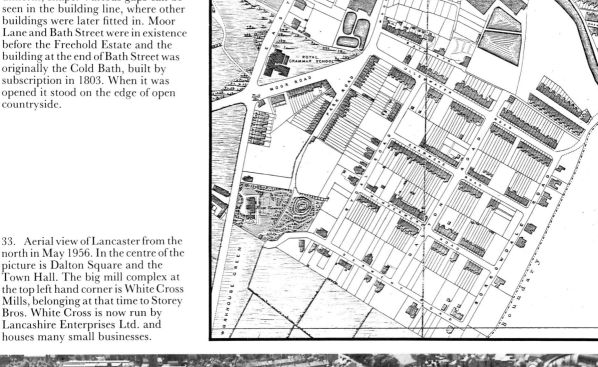

33. Aerial view of Lancaster from the north in May 1956. In the centre of the picture is Dalton Square and the Town Hall. The big mill complex at the top left hand corner is White Cross Mills, belonging at that time to Storey Bros. White Cross is now run by Lancashire Enterprises Ltd. and houses many small businesses.

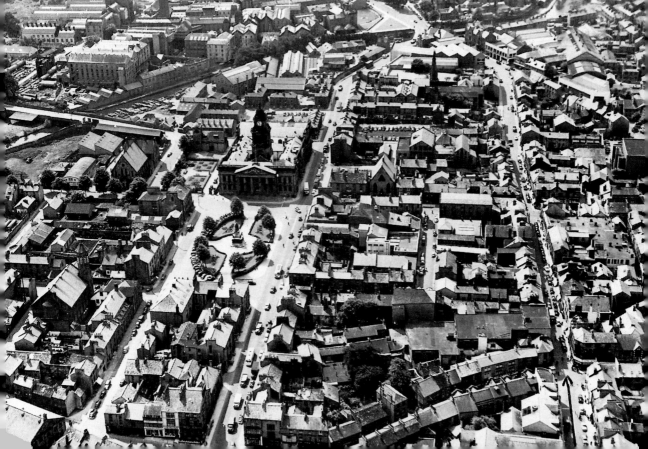

Town Hall
and Market Square

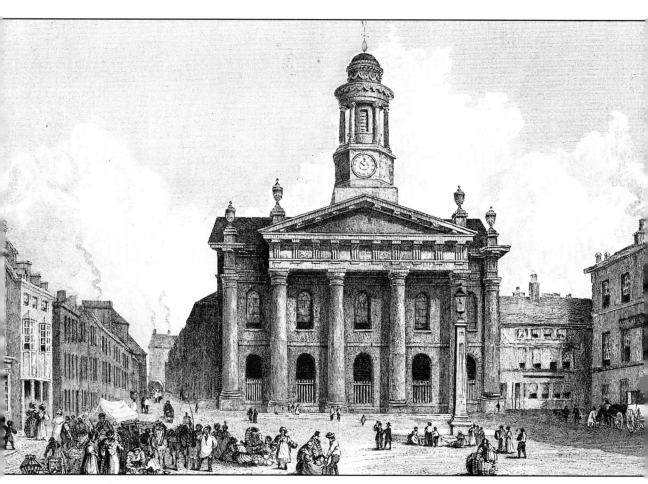

34. The old Town Hall from an engraving by S. Rawle after W. Westall, 1829. The centre of the Market Square has an obelisk in this view, one of many features to have occupied that position. On the right can be seen the *Commercial Inn*, one of the main coaching inns of the late 18th and early 19th centuries.

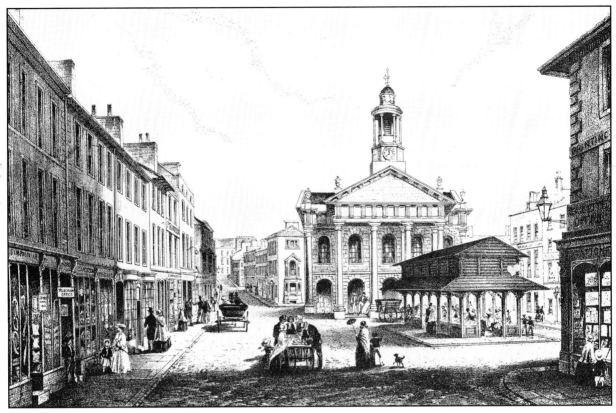

35.   Market Street and the old Town Hall, *c*.1850, from a lithograph by E. H. Buckler. In the Market Square can be seen the wooden market hall built in the 1840s. The Town Hall had at this date an open lower storey serving as a corn exchange.

36.   The old Town Hall, in Market Square, *c*.1900. The ladders leaning against the building on the right belong to the fire brigade. The corporation offices, fire brigade and police were until 1909 all housed in the same building. It is not greatly altered in appearance today, though the urns on the top were removed in the 1950s.

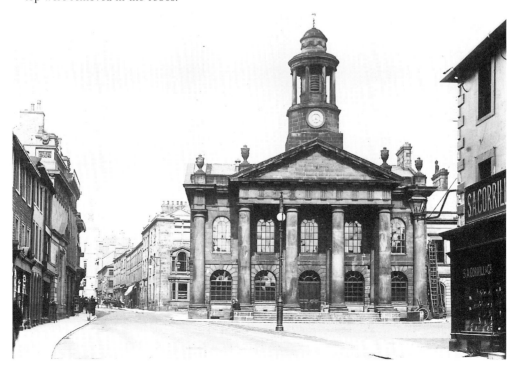

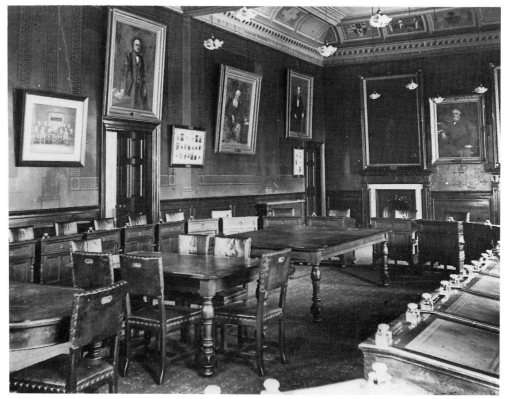

37. The council chamber of the old Town Hall, before 1909. Much of the furniture is by Gillow &
Co., including the committee desks around the edge. The two fireplaces in the end wall are also by
Gillow, dated 1783. This room now forms one of the main display galleries of the City Museum.

38. The Market Square seen from an upper window of the museum in 1973. The view has been totally changed
since pedestrianisation. No longer do buses go up and down the street. The unsightly, if extremely convenient,
public lavatories in the foreground have been replaced by a fountain. Most of the businesses around the Square,
other than the *Blue Anchor*, have changed hands several times since the photograph was taken.

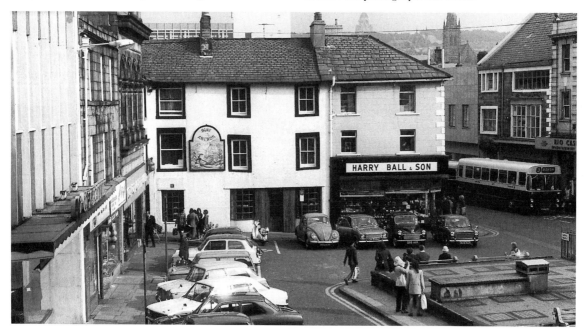

Street Scenes

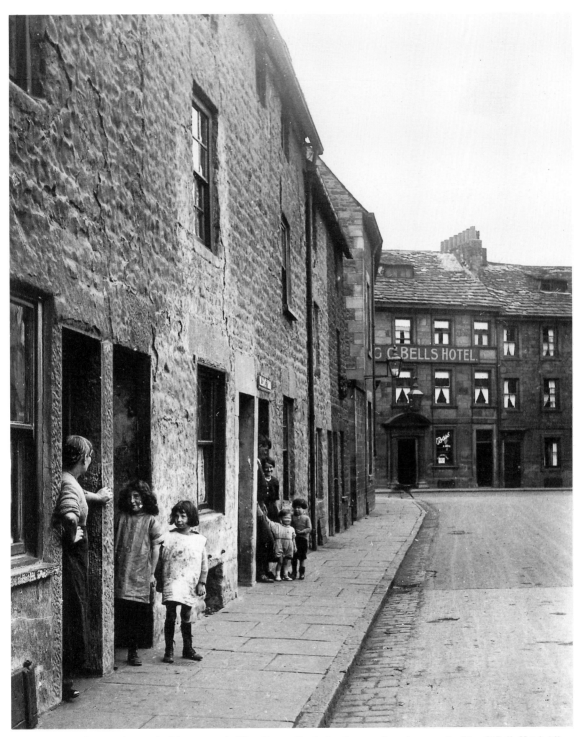

39. Spring Garden Street, looking towards King Street. In the background can be seen the *Ring O'Bells Hotel*. All the houses on the left hand side of the picture have now disappeared. Halfway along the row of houses can be seen the entrance to Wilson's Yard.

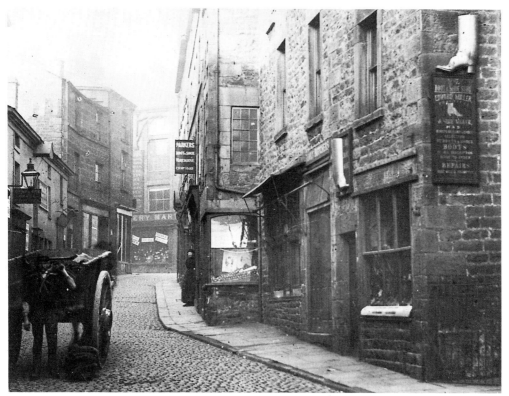

40. View of St Nicholas Street, *c.*1886, looking west. Notice the number of trade signs on the shops. There is a considerable incline between Stonewell at the bottom of the street and Horseshoe Corner at the top. This natural slope is masked by the present shopping centre but represents the original river terrace.

41. St Nicholas Street, looking west. This street, which was a continuation of Market Street, totally disappeared during redevelopment in 1971. It now forms part of the St Nicholas shopping centre and the curving line of the street has been lost.

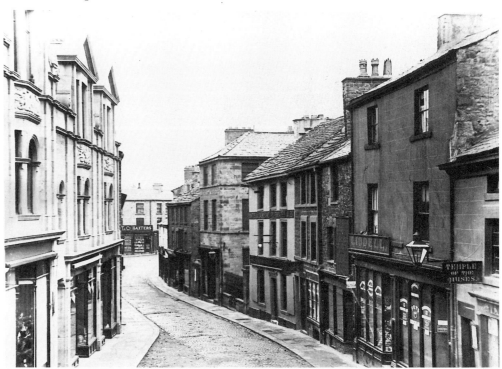

42. Sun Street, looking north in 1927. This was a late addition to the town's street pattern, occupying former gardens behind the *Sun Inn*. In 1797 the land was let out as building lots, and building soon followed. In this area can be seen the Music Room (*see* plates 14 and 15).

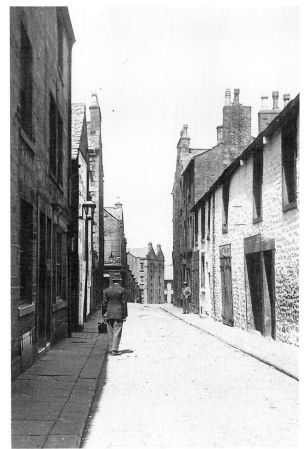

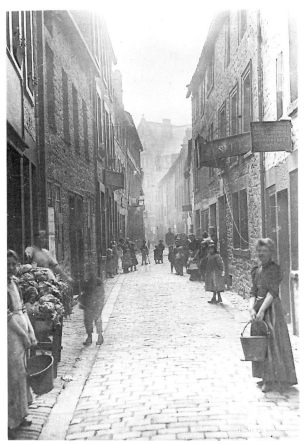

43.· China Lane towards the end of the 19th century. This was one of the poorer parts of the town and many of the houses were lodging houses, which made it very densely populated indeed. China Lane was widened in 1895 and became China Street. It now bears little resemblance to its former self.

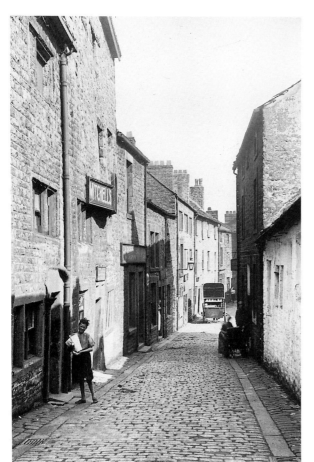

44. Bridge Lane, looking north. Bridge Lane was the main road leading to the bridge over the Lune until Skerton Bridge was built in 1788. The lane itself was very narrow and densely populated by the poorest people in Lancaster. On the left of the picture is the *Carpenters Arms*, a public house formerly known as, and now renamed, the *Three Mariners*. This pub stands on its own in what is left of Bridge Lane, and the whole scene has completely changed.

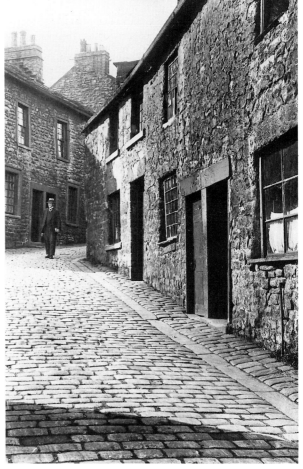

45. Another view of Bridge Lane, looking south. The photograph was taken in about 1927, but apart from the costume of the bystander there is almost nothing to indicate the date.

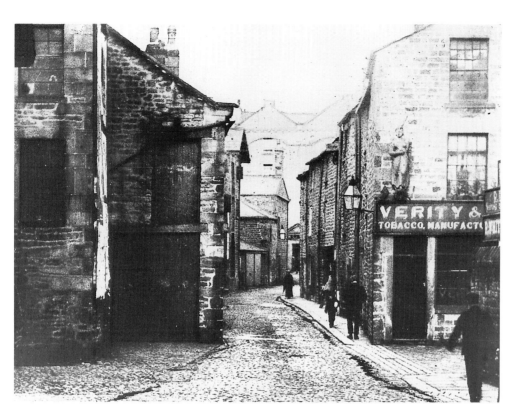

46.   Damside Street in about 1900. Damside Street
followed the line of the medieval mill dam and
probably the original Roman course of the Lune.
From the 18th century it was heavily built up, but
in 1938 virtually the whole area was cleared to build
the bus station. Verity & Co., tobacco
manufacturers, on the right of the picture, have a
carved wooden Red Indian outside, the usual
symbol of their trade.

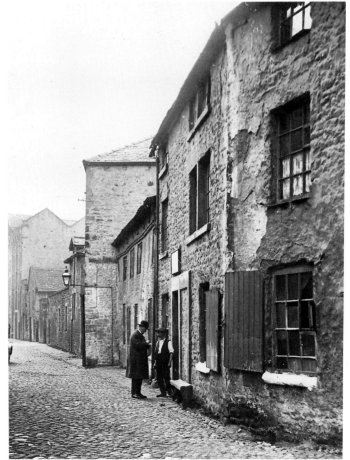

47.   Damside Street, photographed in about 1927.
The poor condition of many of the buildings is
immediately visible. Most have now gone, either for
the building of the bus station in 1938-9 or during
later demolition.

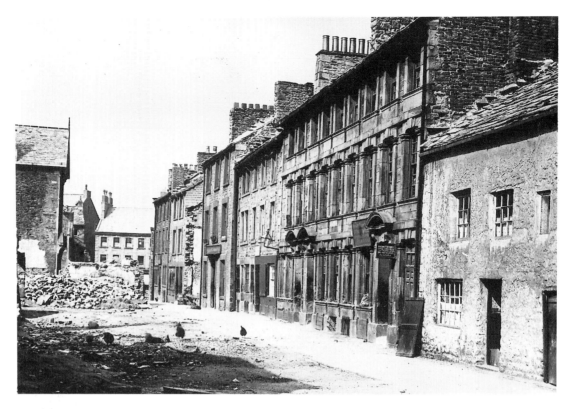

48. China Lane in about 1895. Demolition is under way to widen and change the alignment of this street. In the distance can be seen the narrow gap between the buildings which represents the Church Street end of Bridge Lane.

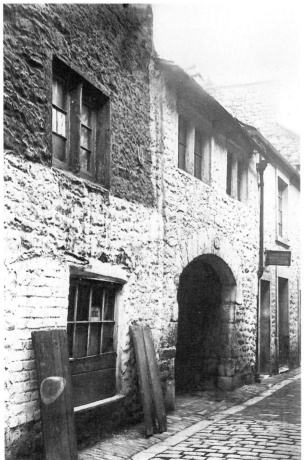

49. Oven House Gates in China Lane. This was a very poor and crowded neighbourhood. The oven house was a communal bake oven where people without access to a stove could have meals cooked.

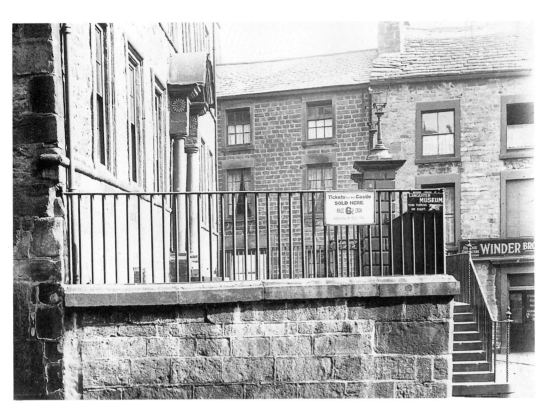

50. The Judges' Lodging in the 1920s. The buildings in the background were demolished many years ago and have been replaced by Mitre House, a Crown building dating from the mid-1970s.

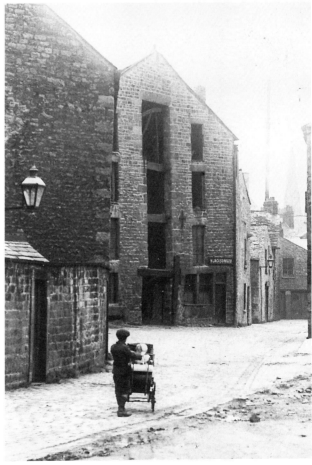

51. Fleet Square, looking towards Damside Street. This area was largely destroyed by the building of the bus station. Both 'Fleet' and 'Damside' are reminders of the ancient millstream which fed the town mill in the Middle Ages.

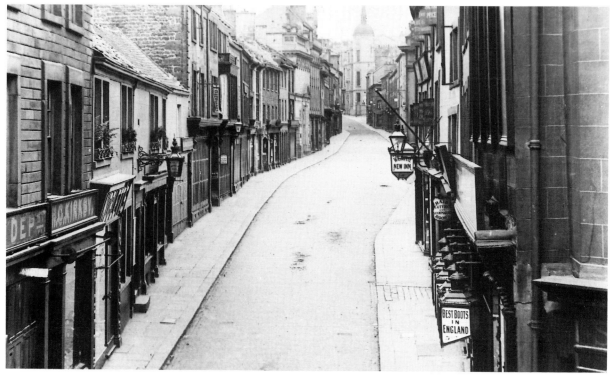

52. Market Street, looking west, around the turn of the century. At the top of the street can be seen the Storey Institute, opened in 1891 and extended in 1906. Most of the shops at this date occupy ancient burgage plots. More recently, plots have been combined for larger shops.

53. James Street in 1927, another crowded thoroughfare. It runs parallel to Penny Street and adjoins the market, but now contains no houses at all.

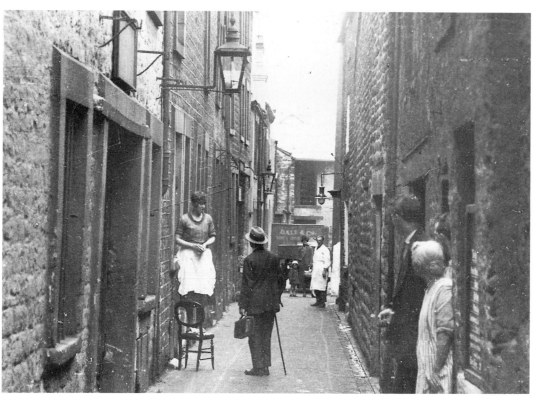

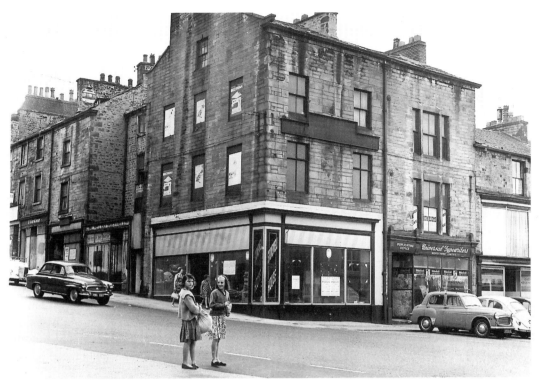

54. Corner of Great John Street and St Nicholas Street from Stonewell, c.1960. This corner was demolished in 1971 to make way for a multi-storey car park and shopping centre.

55. The top end of Penny Street, showing the *Corporation Arms*. The corporation arms (a fleur de lys over a lion passant gardant) were carved in stone over the door of the inn, and are now preserved in the City Museum.

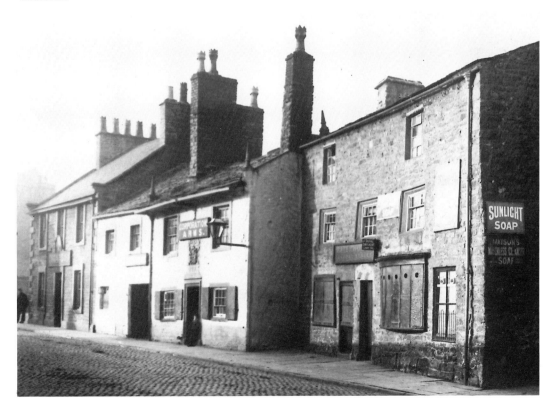

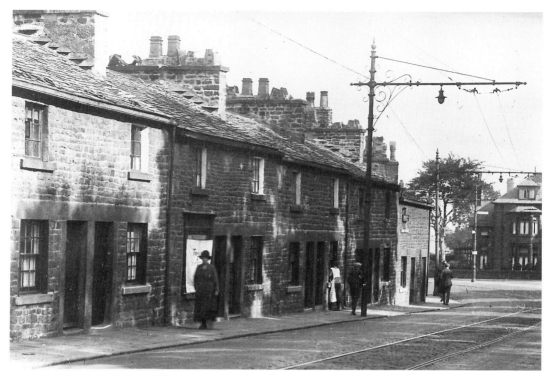

56.   Cottages at the Pointer. The Pointer was a signpost at the junction of Bowerham Road and South Road, which gave its name to these modest houses. Outside can be seen the tramway and tram standards. The area was completely remodelled as a result of major roadworks some years ago, and the houses demolished.

57.   Penny Street Bridge and the *Prince William Henry Hotel*. This was one of the most southerly buildings in Lancaster for many years. Its stable can be seen nearer the bridge. In the field behind many auctions were held, including in 1846 the auction of all the horses used by the Lancaster Canal Co. for pulling its fast packet boats.

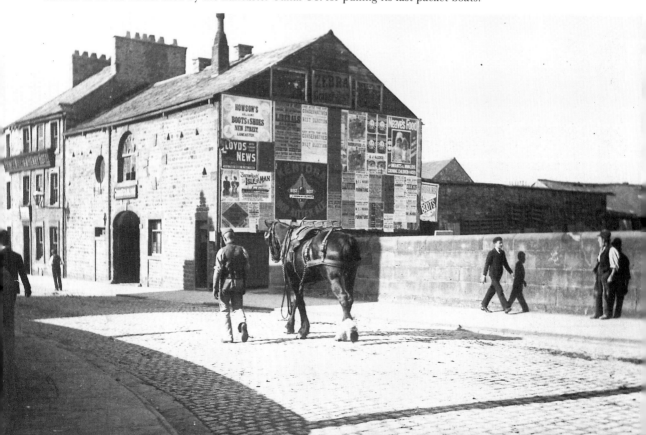

58. St Leonardgate, looking east. In the Middle Ages a leper hospital dedicated to St Leonard lay approximately where the buildings stand in the far distance in the photograph. This was just outside the boundary of Lancaster town, marked by a beck which has since been culverted. To the right lies Factory Hill, where Albion Mill used to stand. The *White Lion Hotel* on the right of the picture was for many years the toll house, where tolls were charged on all goods coming into and out of Lancaster. This was one of three such toll houses.

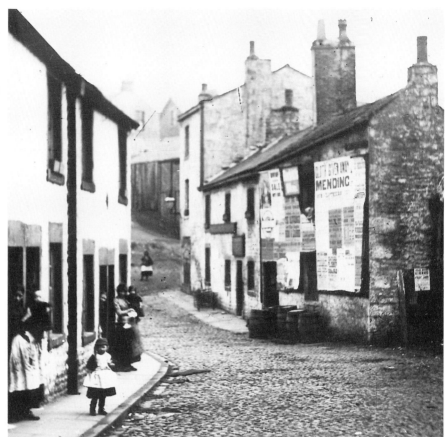

59. St Leonardgate looking west, before the demolition of most of the property in the foreground. On the extreme right is the Grand Theatre, originally built in 1781 but much rebuilt later.

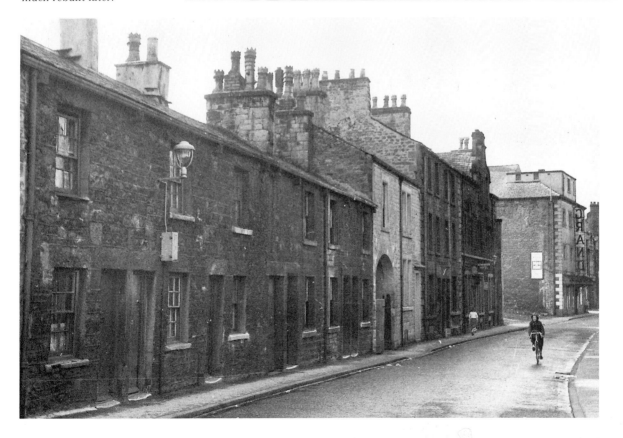

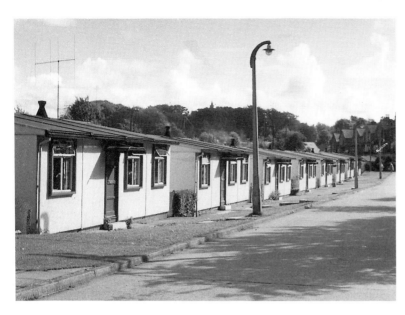

60. Prefabs in Ashton Road. Although these cheap, post-war, and once common houses have now gone, their sites have been occupied by modern houses, the roads and drainage determining their position.

61. The University of Lancaster, seen from the south in 1974. To the right is the M6 motorway and, to the left, the main A6 road. The university occupies the Bailrigg estate between the two roads and about three miles south of Lancaster, which can just be seen in the distance. It was the offer of this large campus which determined the location of the new university in 1963-4. The most prominent buildings are the Chaplaincy Centre (top left) and Bowland Tower (centre), which occupies a corner of Alexandra Square. The university is built along a pedestrian spine, which runs north-south, while servicing is carried out from perimeter roads.

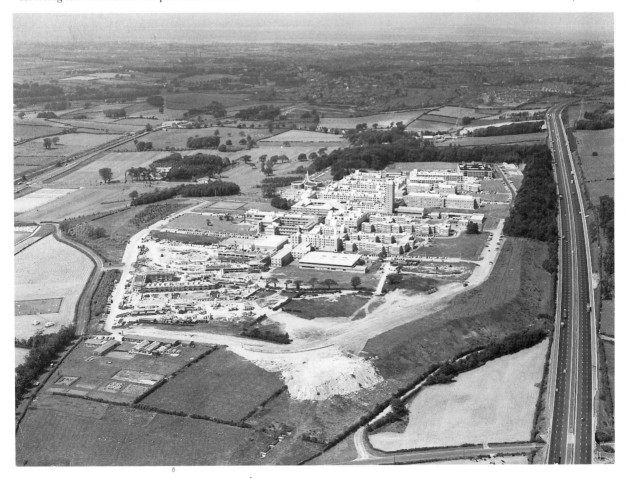

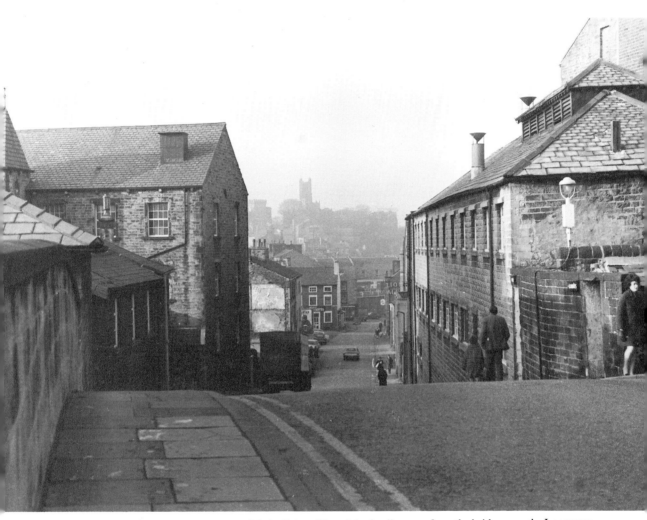

62. Moor Lane, 1973. The view is to the east with the Priory Church in the distance, from the bridge over the Lancaster Canal. The mills on either side of the lane, Moor Lane Mills North and South, had a varied career. Moor Lane Mills South began before 1825 as a sailcloth manufactory. Both mills came into the hands of William Storey in 1861, and were used for cotton spinning.

Yards and Courts

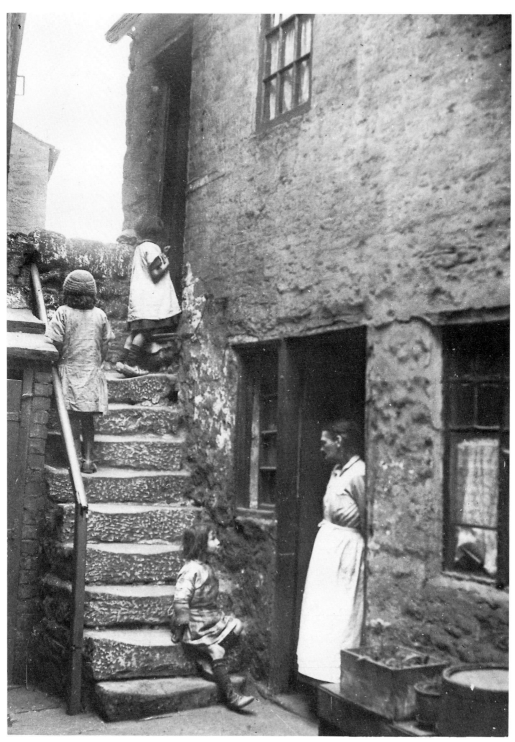

63. Bolton's Yard, off Spring Garden Street. Typical of many slum tenements, the houses were divided into several levels and approached by steps. Probably each family rented only one room.

64. Atkinson's Yard, Market Street, during demolition on 11 April 1894. The yard took its name from Atkinson's watchmakers, which occupied the frontage. Like many of the yards which housed such a large part of the urban population, it lay very close to the town centre and was approached through archways such as the one in the foreground.

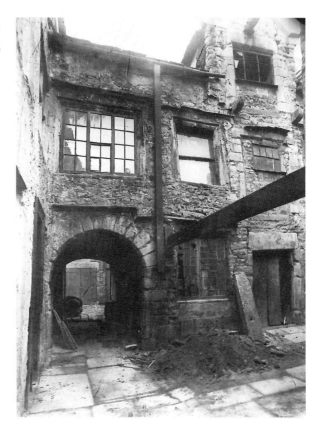

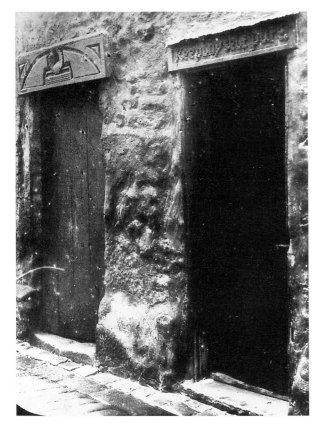

65. Bridge Lane: houses in Albert Square. Albert Square was a small 1850s' development perched above Bridge Lane and below the Vicarage Field. During the building of the houses a Roman coin hoard was discovered. The door lintel on the right, reading 'Keep thyself pure', is carved out of wood and is now in Lancaster City Museum.

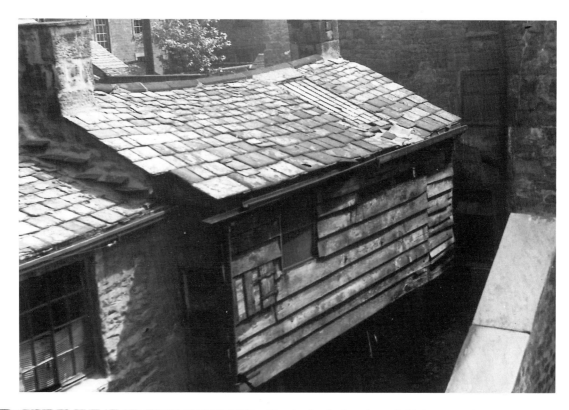

66. An intriguing piece of old Lancaster is this wooden structure in Horse and Farrier Yard, off Brock Street. It is thought to have served as a theatre where travelling players performed, but nothing survives of it now.

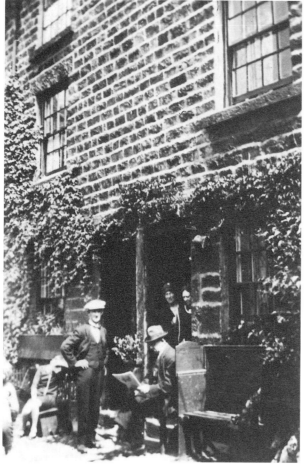

67. Riley's Yard on the south side of Common Garden Street. The entrance was opposite the end of James Street.

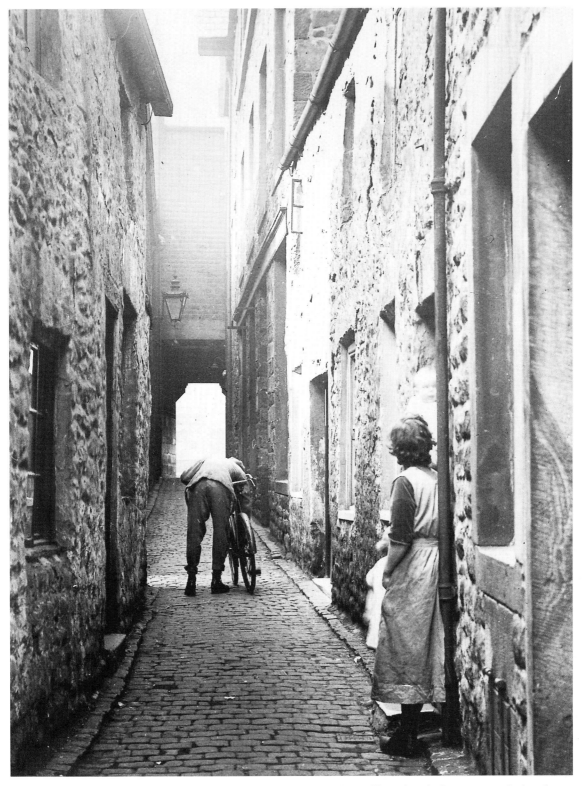

68.   Off to work. A view in Chancery Lane, taken about 1927. The lane still survives, its future uncertain, but there are now no houses on it at all. This lane, with Anchor Lane, forms a short cut between Market Street and Church Street. The houses in both lanes were small cramped buildings with no rear access, cellars or foundations.

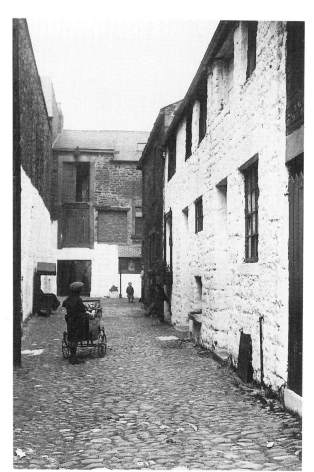

69. Barrow's Yard, off Cornmarket Street. Typical of many of the yards, this one has whitewashed buildings to increase the light, and a communal water supply. Cornmarket Street now forms the western approach to the market, behind King Street. The yard has totally disappeared.

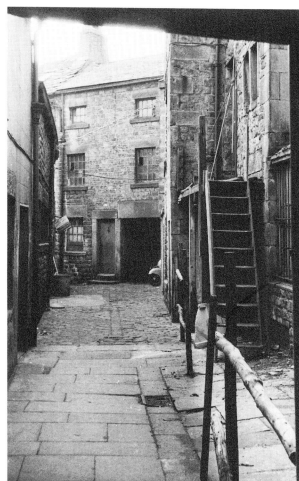

70. Bashful Alley, linking Market Street and King Street, photographed about 1962. Despite the late date the atmosphere is very much of the 19th century except for the motor scooter just appearing at the end of the alley. There is no explanation of the origin of the name, but in the 18th century it was different – and unprintable.

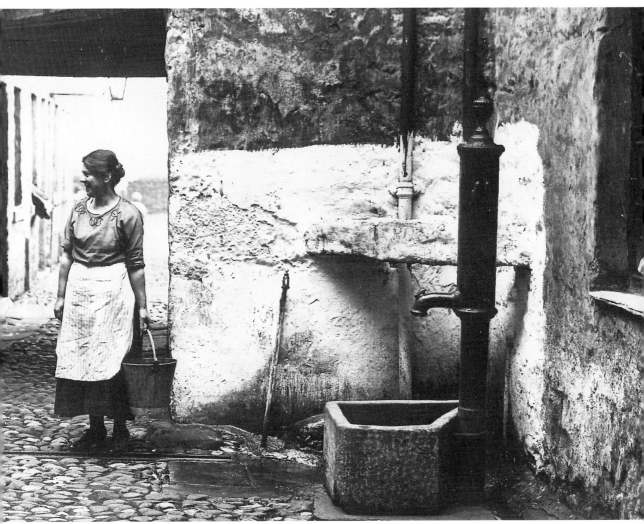

71. St Mary's Place, a typical Lancaster yard, much photographed because of its picturesque nature. Here is the communal water supply. St Mary's Place lay off St Mary Gate, at the top end of Church Street, immediately below the Priory Church.

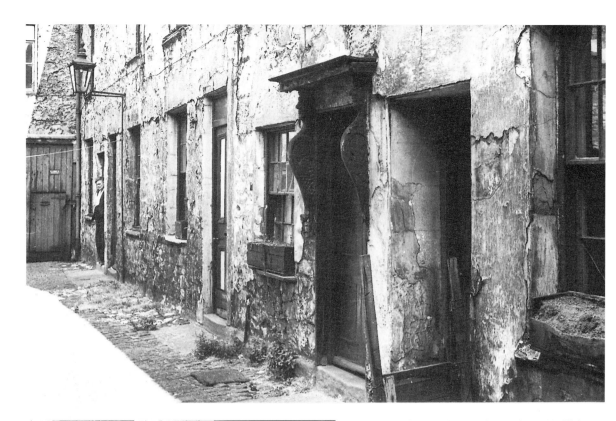

72. King's Place, off King Street, in 1960. This surprisingly late survival of a once common type of yard is very striking. Particularly noticeable are the elaborate door surrounds of the house at the centre, which look as though they have been 'borrowed' from a rather grander building.

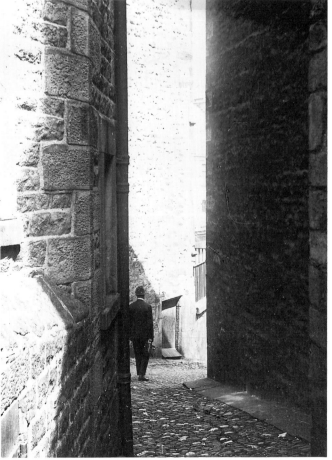

73. Nip Hill, one of the useful little byways linking main streets, in this case Church Street and Castle Hill. In the background is the corner of the Judges' Lodging.

Shops and Signs

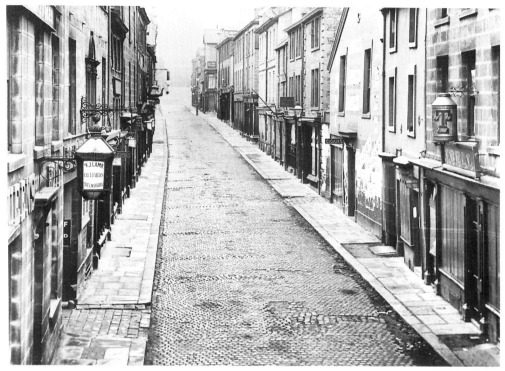

74. Penny Street, looking south. A fine array of shop signs can be seen, including the large tinplate kettle (far left) over T. D. Smith's grocer's shop and (right) the golden canister over John R. & W. Bell Ltd. Both these shop signs are now in the City Museum.

75. A closer view of the golden canister in situ on its shop.

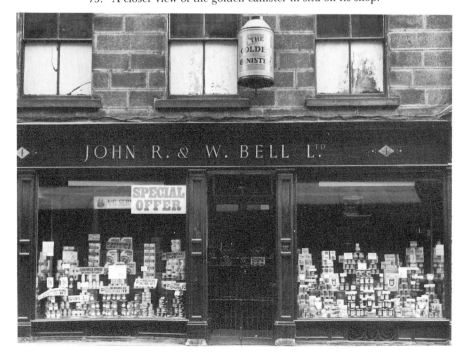

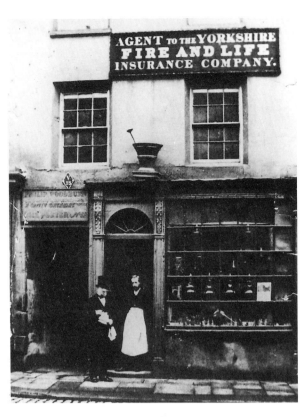

76. (*Left*) Whimpray & Cardwell in Market Street, photographed in 1880. The pestle and mortar symbol of a chemist is a feature of this shop. Another, moved in 1985 from Market Street, can now be seen on a chemist's shop in New Street.

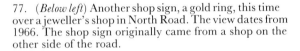

77. (*Below left*) Another shop sign, a gold ring, this time over a jeweller's shop in North Road. The view dates from 1966. The shop sign originally came from a shop on the other side of the road.

78. (*Below*) Lawson's toy shop in New Street. The shop was established in 1837 and a rocking horse has been used as its sign ever since. From time to time sections of the horse are replaced, and it is unlikely that any part of the present horse is original.

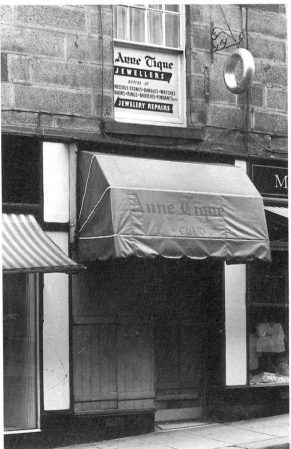

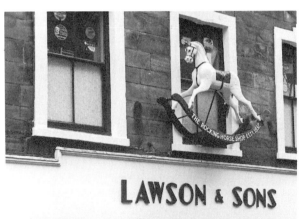

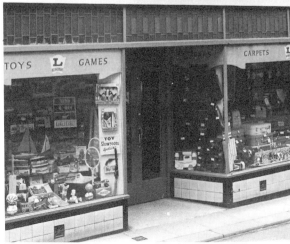

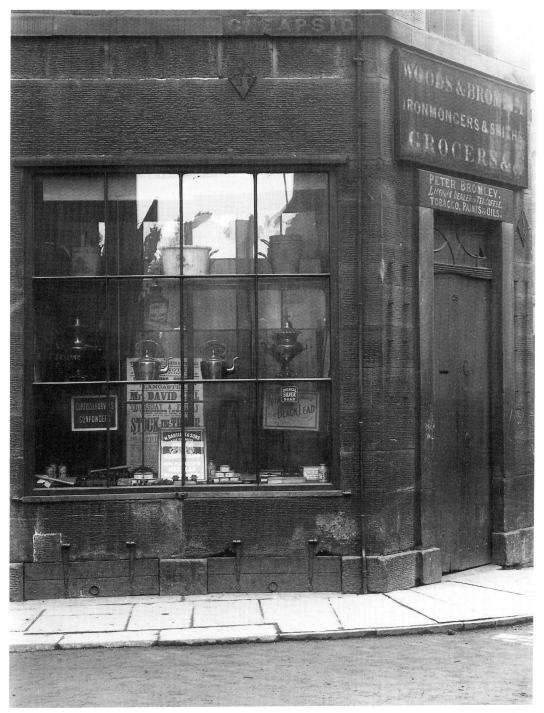

79. The shop of Woods & Bromley, ironmongers and grocers at Horseshoe Corner from *c*.1844 to 1900. The window display is very modest compared with many, and the photograph does not seem to have been taken for advertising purposes as was frequently the case, when rather more crowded windows and elaborate displays were normal.

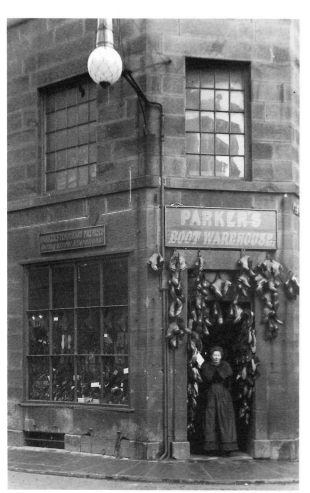

80. Parker's Boot Warehouse on the corner of Cheapside and St Nicholas Street. Note the fine display of boots outside. This shop appears in plate 79 as the premises of Woods & Bromley, ironmongers. This junction is known as Horseshoe Corner from the horseshoe set in the roadway. It probably marks the site of a horse fair.

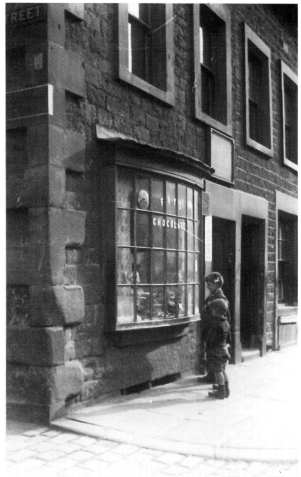

81. A tempting display: a grocer's shop at the corner of Cable Street and Wood Street in the 1920s. This area was demolished to make way for the bus station in 1939.

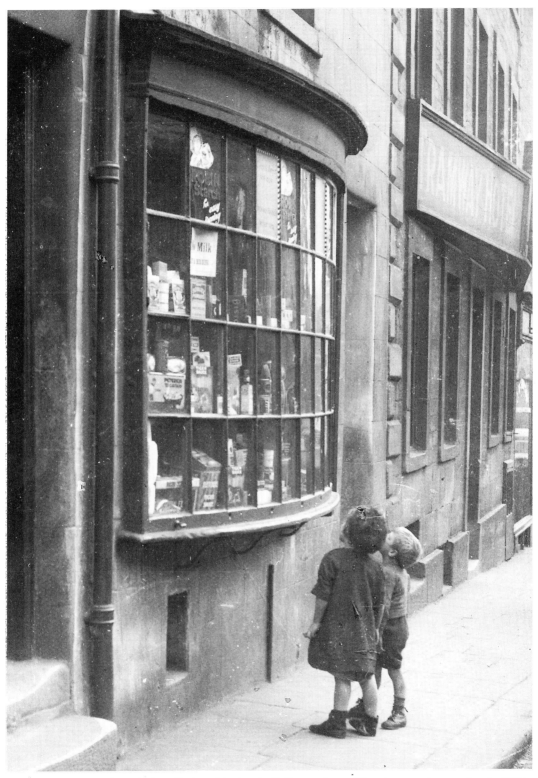

82. Another tempting window display, this time in St Leonardgate. The photograph was taken in 1927.

The Castle

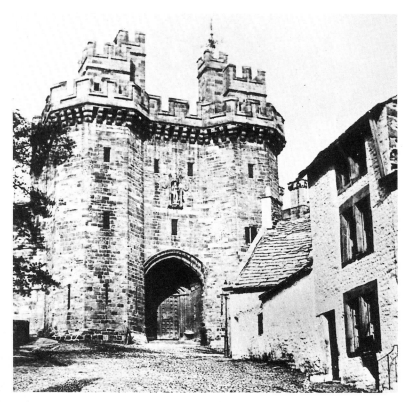

83. The castle gateway, *c.*1875. Cottages lined what had once been the castle moat and obstructed the view of the gatehouse. In one of these cottages by the castle gate the artist Cornelius Henderson was born, and his father, John Henderson, an amateur artist, pursued the trade of shoemaker. In 1876 a subscription was raised to demolish the buildings and improve the view of the castle, and this was accordingly done.

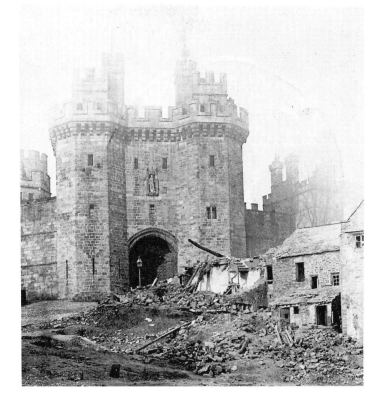

84. The castle gateway in 1876, following the demolition of cottages which stood in front of it.

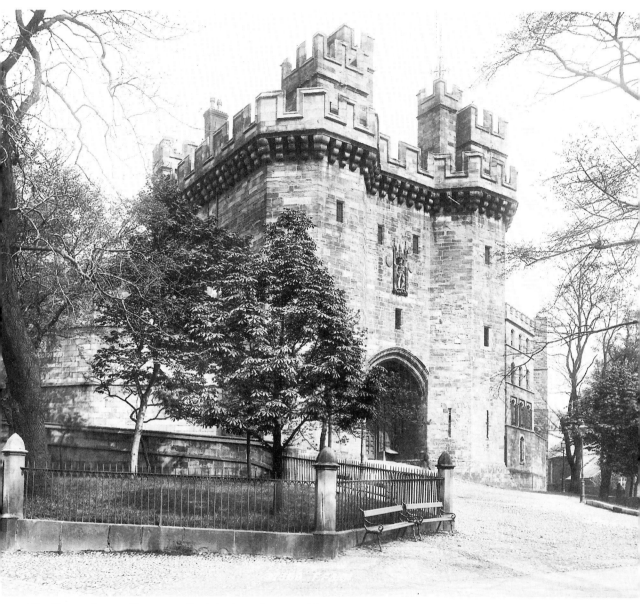

85. The gatehouse of Lancaster Castle in the early years of the 20th century, long before the railings were removed. The railed areas to both left and right of the gatehouse represent the original line of the moat, long since filled in.

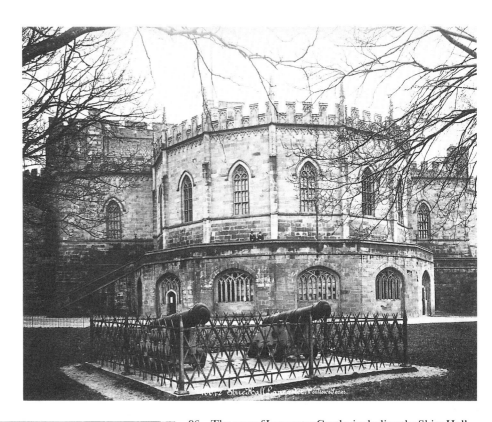

86. The rear of Lancaster Castle, including the Shire Hall. The pair of guns in the foreground, protected by a spiked fence, were captured in the Crimea. They were removed for scrap in 1941, along with the railings, but the stone plinth on which they stood still remains. This is believed to cover the graves of the 20 persons executed in 1817.

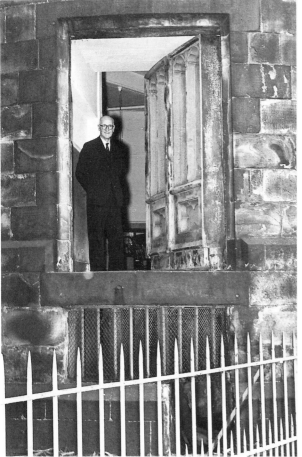

87. The hanging door at Hanging Corner at the rear of the castle, open for repairs in 1962. Until 1865 executions were carried out in public on a scaffold at this point.

Churches

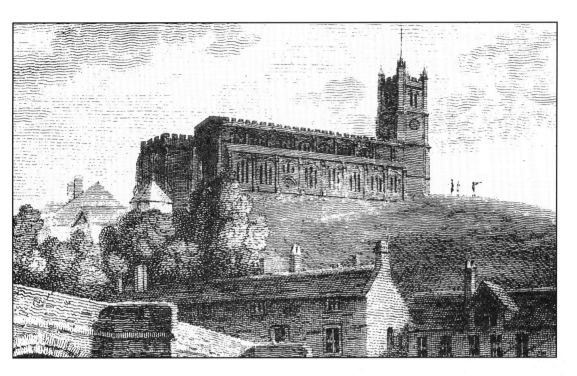

88. The Priory Church, from an engraving of 1797. This view illustrates well the splendid commanding position and the length of the building. The west tower was added in 1754 to replace an earlier structure which stood slightly detached from the church. The new tower made a marvellous leading mark for ships coming up the river.

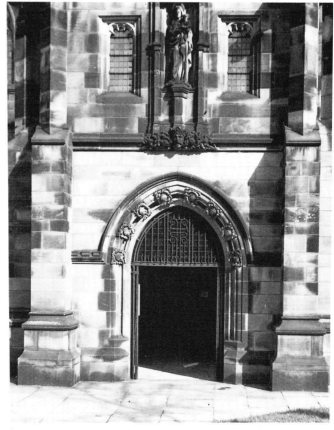

89. The south porch of Lancaster Priory Church, added in 1903 by the local firm, Paley & Austin. This splendid piece of architecture replaces an earlier porch of 1816. It was designed by Hubert Austin and given in memory of Jacob Pearson Langshaw and his wife Emily by their daughter Fanny Austin, wife of the architect.

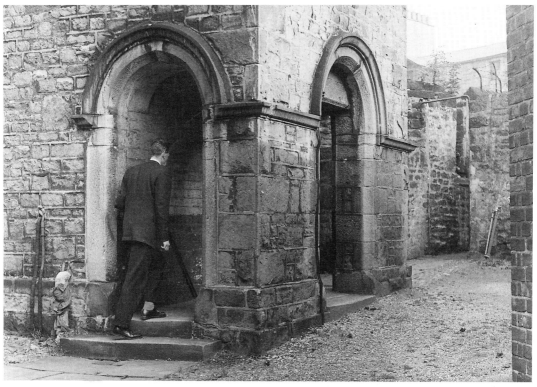

90. Entrance to the Presbyterian chapel in St Nicholas Street. The chapel was built in 1787 by Thomas Taylor, and could seat about 300 people.

91. St Peter's Church, built by Paley & Austin and now the Roman Catholic cathedral for the diocese of Lancaster. The buildings were completed in 1859 at a cost of £12,000.

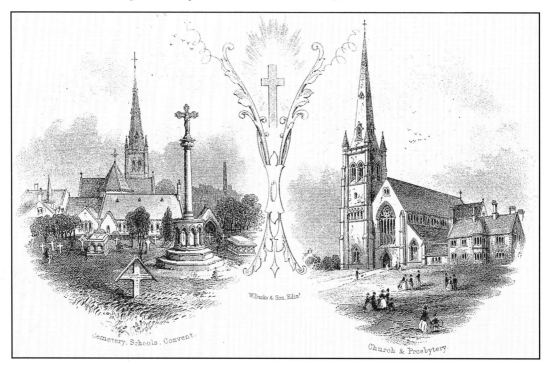

92. Chapel Street at the turn of the century, looking towards St John's Church. The tramlines in the foreground were used by the Lancaster and District tramways, which were horse-drawn from beginning to end. The area on which Chapel Street and St John's itself stand was originally part of the Green Ayre, an island lying to the south of the river and defined by the millstream. Most of the buildings in this area date from the mid-18th century, when it started to be developed.

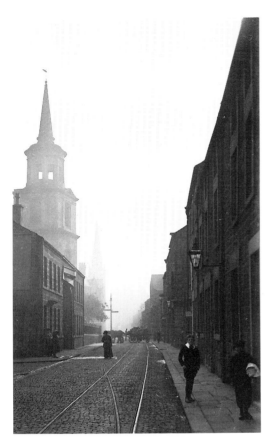

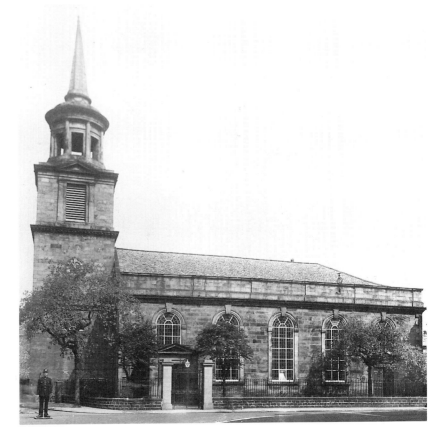

93. St John's Church. The church itself was built in 1755 on Green Ayre at a place known as the Clay Holes. The architect is unknown. The tower was added some 30 years later by the architect Thomas Harrison, under the will of John Bowes, a Lancaster merchant. The whole church is a magnificent example of Georgian building, with relatively few alterations and additions. The church became redundant in 1981 and is now maintained by the Redundant Churches Fund. This photograph is from a presentation album to a former vicar in the 1930s.

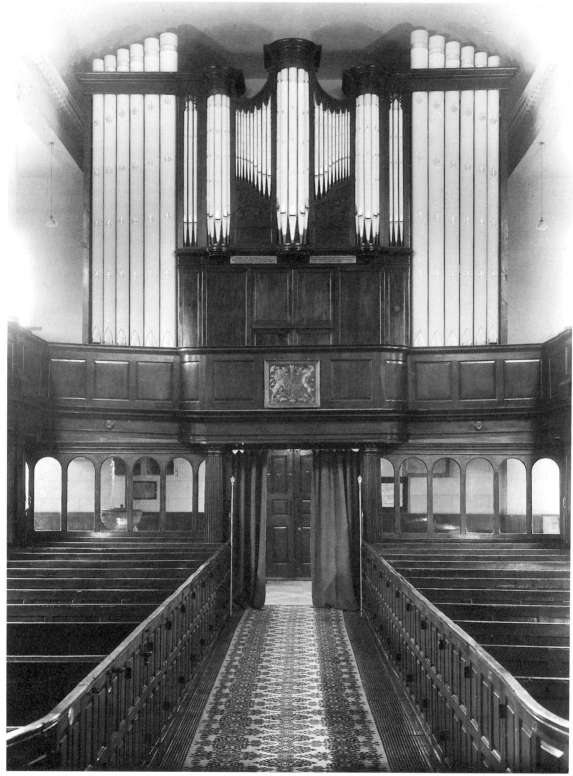

94. The interior of St John's Church, looking west, showing the box pews and the magnificent screen and organ. The organ was built by the local firm of Langshaw, but has been much extended at various times until it now fills the whole gallery. Most pews were owned by individual families, but a large double pew on the south side was for many years the Corporation pew. In the early days of the church it was the custom for members of the Corporation to go to church at Lancaster Priory on Sunday morning and to St John's in the afternoon.

Other Buildings

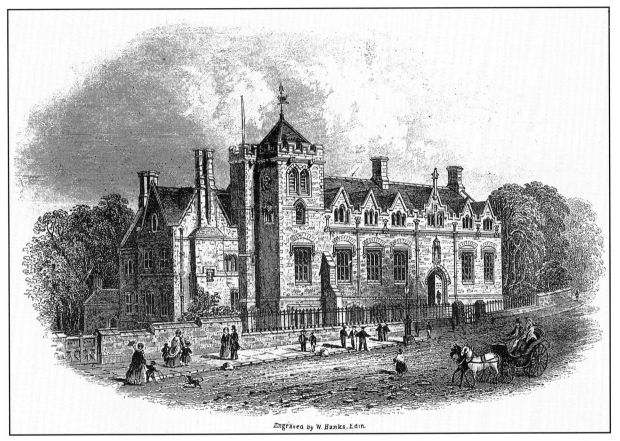

Engraved by W. Banks, Edin.

95. Lancaster Royal Grammar School on East Road. The school was originally established close to the Priory Church but outgrew its site by the mid-19th century. The new buildings were designed by Edmund Sharp and E. G. Paley in 1851-5. There has been considerable further building since then on both sides of East Road.

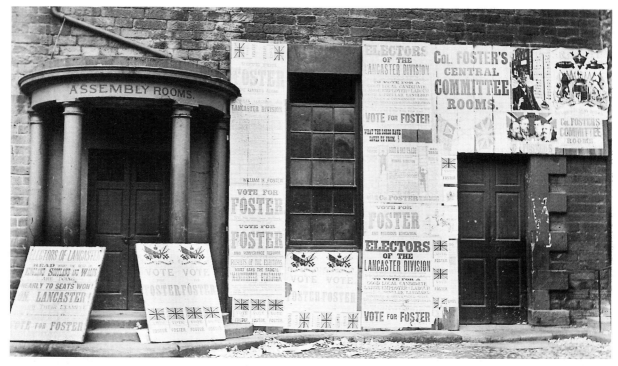

96.   The Assembly Room in King Street, in use here as Colonel Foster's committee rooms during the 1895 elections. Colonel Foster, who lived at Hornby Castle, was the Conservative candidate, and was also the proprietor of Queensbury Mills in Yorkshire, better known as Black Dyke Mills.

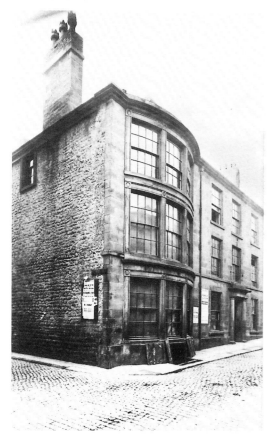

97.   The old *King's Arms Hotel*, before demolition and rebuilding in 1879. Many travellers refer to its magnificent interior and great bow windows. It was for centuries the premier inn of Lancaster. It had clearly started life as a smaller building to which others were added as time went on, leading to a rather curious polygonal site at the junction of King Street and Meeting House Lane. Among its many visitors Charles Dickens, who came here in 1857, is probably one of the most famous.

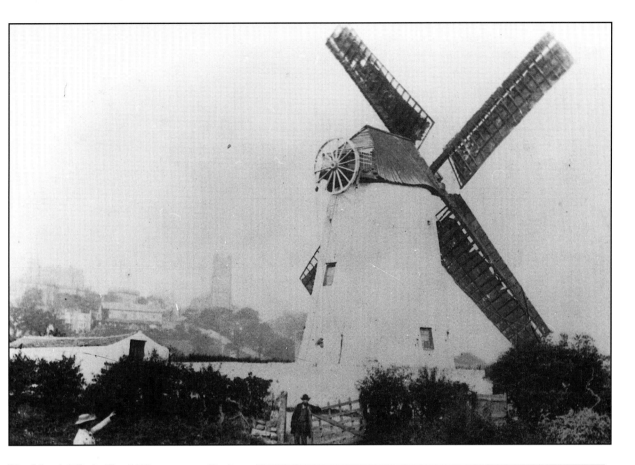

98. Marsh Windmill, *c.*1870, a tower mill of stone which was long a landmark of Lancaster standing near the junction of Willow Lane and West Road. It was demolished in 1880 by Lancaster Corporation. Other windmills had formerly existed at Scotforth and on Lancaster Moor.

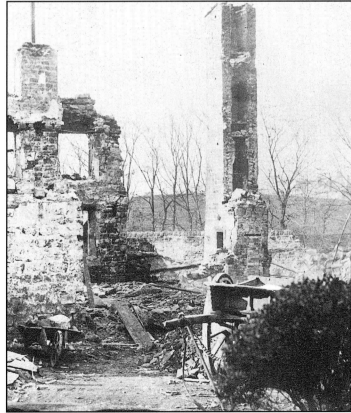

99. White Cross Mills after the fire in 1861. White Cross Mills was singularly unfortunate in the number of serious fires it sustained during the 19th century. The photograph was taken by J. L. Whalley.

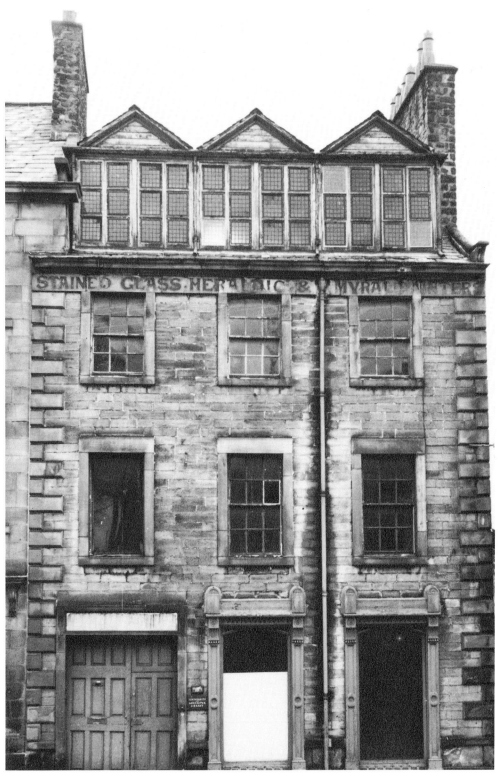

100.   The studios of Shrigley & Hunt, Castle Hill. This was one of Lancaster's numerous firms of stained glass manufacturers, working on many churches and also on private houses. The large windows on the top floor were to light the design studio.

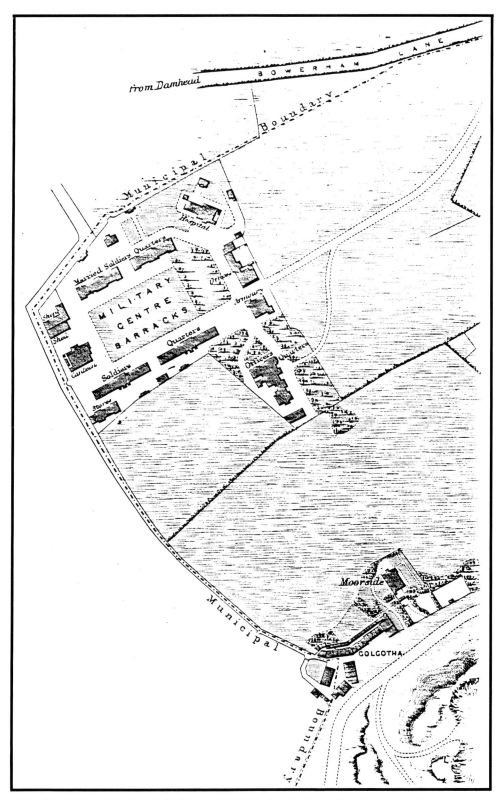

101. Detail from Harrison & Hall's map of 1877, showing Bowerham Barracks, then under construction. The Square has now been built over, but many of the original buildings survive. The whole complex has been used since 1964 as St Martin's College, a teacher training college. To the north-east of the barracks lies Golgotha Village, a terrace of small houses for workers at the town quarries, now marked by Williamson Park.

Lord Ashton

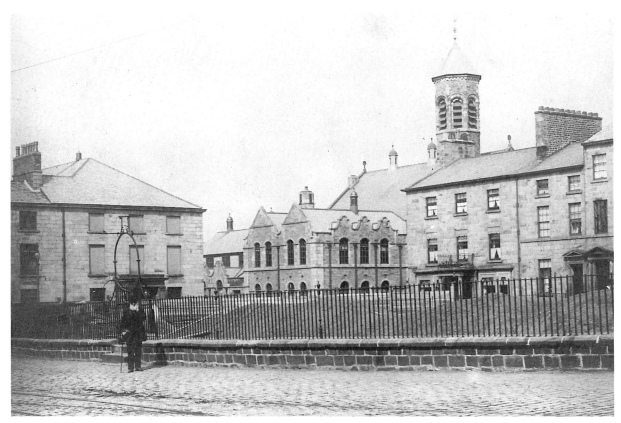

102.   Dalton Square, seen from the west, *c.*1908. The original railings and oval enclosures were replaced in 1908 by the statue of Queen Victoria and the present stone-balustraded oval. To the left of the picture can be seen Palatine Hall, built in 1798 as the first purpose-built Roman Catholic church in Lancaster. It now forms offices for Lancaster City Council.

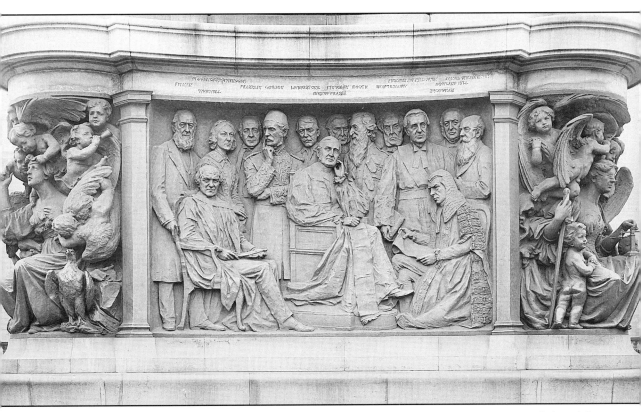

103. The Queen Victoria monument in Dalton Square, given by Lord Ashton in 1908. On the base appear relief portraits in bronze of eminent Victorians. Among these the donor placed his father, James Williamson, who can be seen at the far right, with a beard.

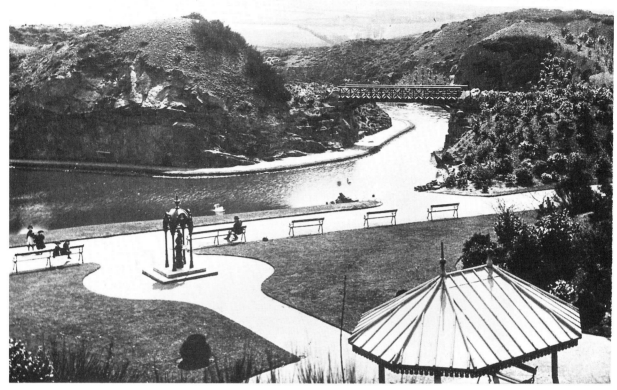

104. Early days in Williamson Park, before 1904. The rocks underlying the park planting can be seen and the park shows its quarry origins very clearly. The rustic bridge in the middle distance was later replaced by a stone bridge.

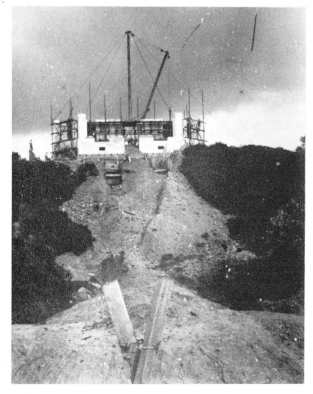

105. The Ashton Memorial under construction in 1906-7. This snapshot view, taken by a former member of the City Museum staff while a boy, using simple equipment, seems to be the only surviving photograph showing the construction. The mass of earth and stone in the foreground is now the site of the grand staircase. The building, apparently of stone construction, is in fact stone cladding on structural steel and concrete. This mixture caused severe problems after a few years and necessitated a complete restoration in 1986-7.

106.   Bronze medal issued on the occasion of the opening of the new Town Hall in 1909. The Town Hall was one of Lord Ashton's benefactions, and it was intended that he should carry out the official opening on 22 December. However, his illness and a period of bad weather caused the postponement of the opening to 27 December. Copies of medals with both dates are in existence. Bronze medals were handed out, along with boxes of chocolates, to all schoolchildren in Lancaster at the time, and also to various dignitaries. Silver medals were struck for V.I.P.s.

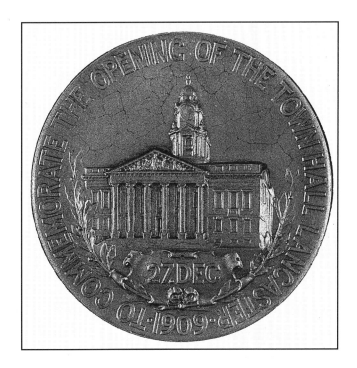

107.   The new Town Hall, complete but not yet opened in 1909. Lord Ashton gave it to the people of Lancaster when the old Town Hall became too small. The Corporation could not afford the cost of a new building itself; this one cost £155,000. Like many public buildings of the period it was intended to dominate and to impress, and it certainly achieves its purpose. The building contract was won by the firm of Gillow & Co., who also carried out most of the magnificent wooden panelling and the internal furnishing.

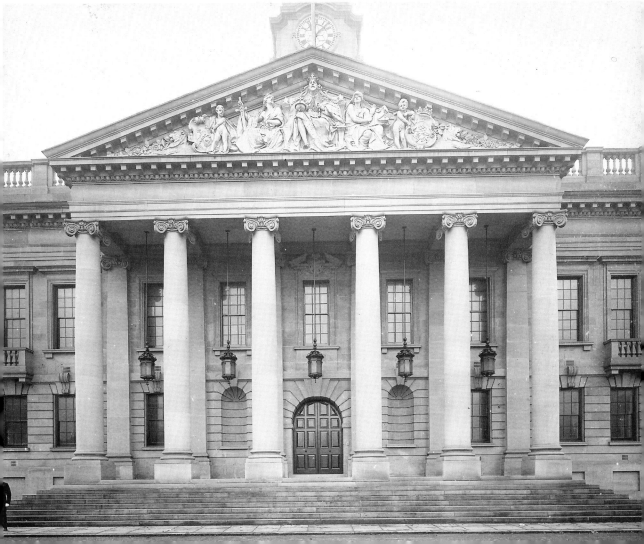

Bridges and the Canal

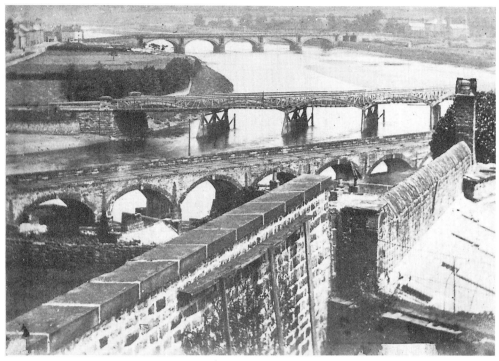

108. A row of bridges. This view, taken from the summer house at the rear of Grey Court in St Marygate, shows three of Lancaster's bridges in 1861. In the foreground is the railway bridge which carried the line from Green Ayre Station to Castle Station. Behind it is the timber Greyhound Bridge, which carried the line from Green Ayre to Morecambe. This bridge was later rebuilt in steel. In the far distance can be seen the grand Skerton Bridge of 1788, designed by Thomas Harrison.

109. Looking back across Greyhound Bridge towards the Priory Church. Photograph by J.L. Whalley, 1861.

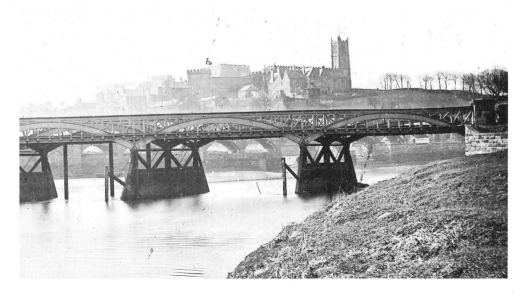

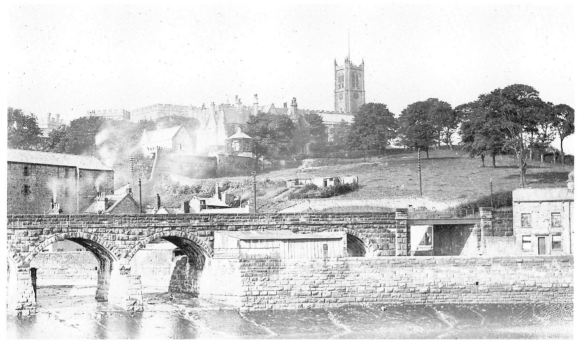

110. The view across the River Lune towards the Priory Church, showing the railway bridge carrying the line from Green Ayre Station to Glasson Dock and the Castle Station. Vicarage Fields can be seen in the background.

111. The splendid Lune Aqueduct carrying the Lancaster Canal over the River Lune above Lancaster. The aqueduct, built by John Rennie and Alexander Stevens, cost £48,000 and was completed in 1797. During construction steam engines were used for pile driving, a very early use of mechanisation on a canal. The aqueduct was clearly designed to be the showpiece of the Canal Company, and consumed so much money that a corresponding aqueduct at Preston could never be built.

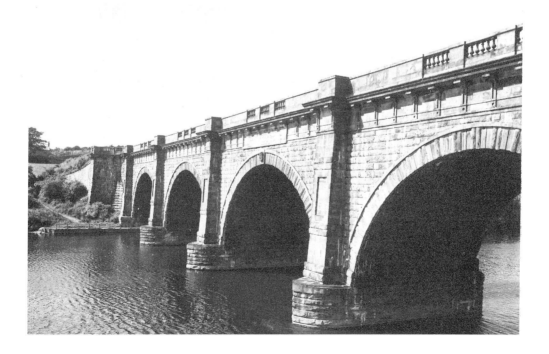

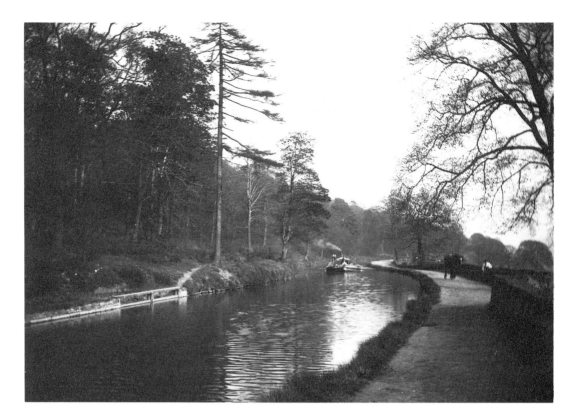

112. A peaceful scene on the Lancaster Canal, with a horse-drawn barge. The canal is no longer used for industrial purposes but is a popular venue for leisure pursuits. It has tremendous potential for development, but the utmost care is needed to preserve its peaceful atmosphere and appearance.

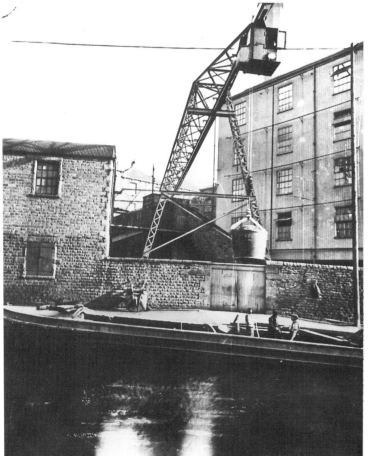

113. Delivery of coal at Storey's White Cross Mill, c.1947. The coal was delivered by barge and was lifted by a gantry placed across the canal. The positioning of most of Lancaster's mills by the canal reflected not only their access to coal supplies, but also the availability of flat building land on the edge of the town.

Shipping and the Quay

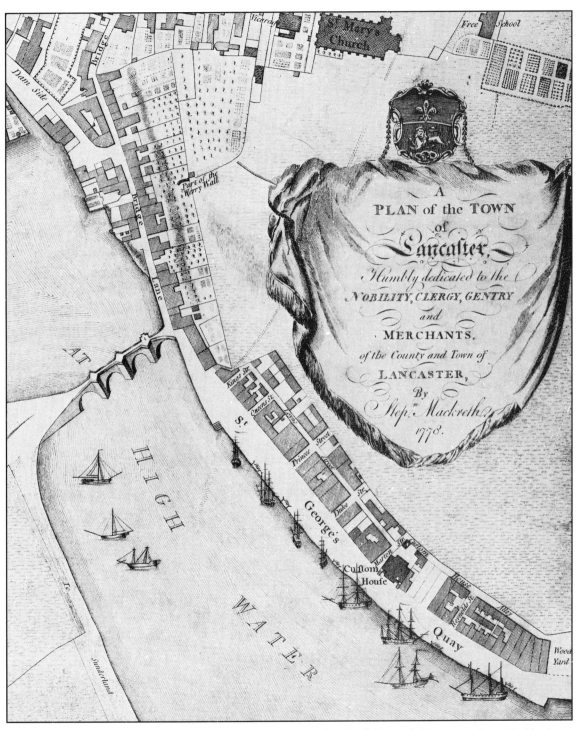

114. A detail from Stephen Mackreth's map of Lancaster, 1778, showing St George's Quay, complete with shipping in the Lune and the old bridge. At this time the large warehouses adjacent to the Custom House to the west did not yet exist. The back streets provided housing for a number of poor people and for those, such as cartmen, whose employment was on the Quay.

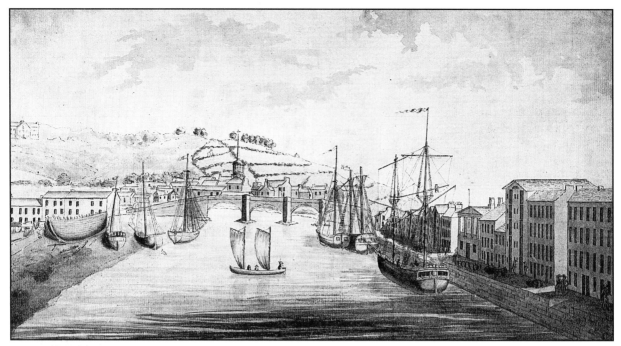

115. St George's Quay looking towards the old bridge, probably around 1790. On the right can be seen some of the warehouses and the Custom House, which the artist has drawn somewhat inaccurately. Behind the bridge is St John's church tower, and on the hill to the extreme left is the workhouse, built in 1788. Below it can be seen Smith's shipyard, with a ship being built. The ship against the quay near the bridge has been 'rigged down', a practice common in the days of hemp rope, when top masts and rigging were sent down during any lengthy stay in port. The picture seems to be unfinished as there is no view of the castle or Priory Church to the right.

116. The Carlisle Bridge over the Lune seen through the rigging of ships lying at Ford Quay. The bridge was built in 1846 and rebuilt in 1866, after this photograph was taken.

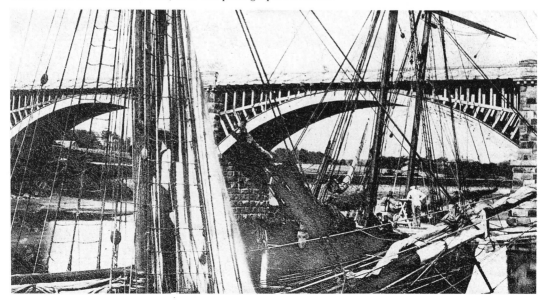

117. Detail from an engraving after J. C. Ibbotson of Lancaster from Cable Street. On the right can be seen a ship under construction at Brockbank's shipyard on the Green Ayre. Ships built at this time had to be floated through the old bridge and fitted out downstream. After 1802, when the first arch of the old bridge was pulled down, ships could be fitted out above the bridge.

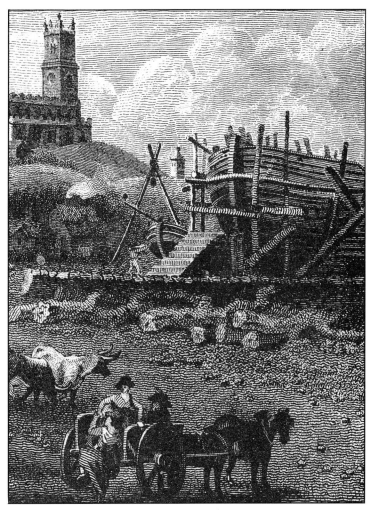

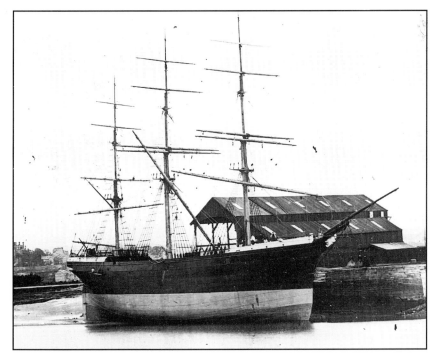

118. The ship *Wennington* at the New Quay in 1865. *Wennington*, a three-masted ship of iron construction, was the first to be built by the Lune Shipbuilding Company. She can be seen here at low tide after launching and during her fitting out. The company built 14 fine vessels.

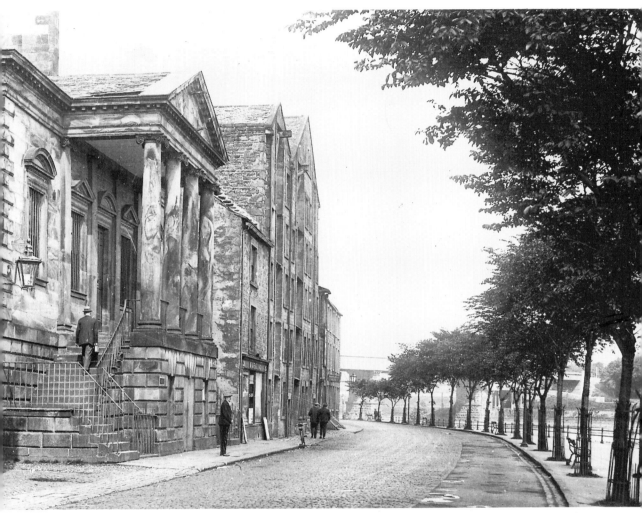

119. St George's Quay and the Custom House, *c.*1927. The Custom House now forms Lancaster's Maritime Museum, opened in 1985. Its stone columns came from Mainstones Quarry at Ellel, and cost five guineas in 1764. The shop next door has now gone, but the warehouses have in recent years been converted to offices and housing.

120. Warehouse on St George's Quay, its main doorway flanked by cannons. These have long since disappeared in wartime scrap drives, but were probably used to protect the steps from the wheels of carts. Over the door are the remains of sign-writing reading 'London Porter'.

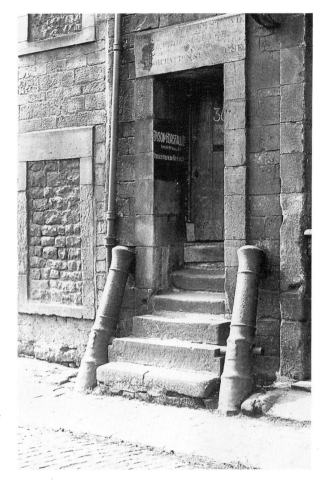

121. Dinghy racing on the Lune, c.1890-1900. The railway line in the foreground ran to Morecambe. In the background is Ford Quay, the second of Lancaster's main quays on the river, and behind it is the monumental St George's Works. To the left is Carlisle Bridge, as rebuilt in 1866.

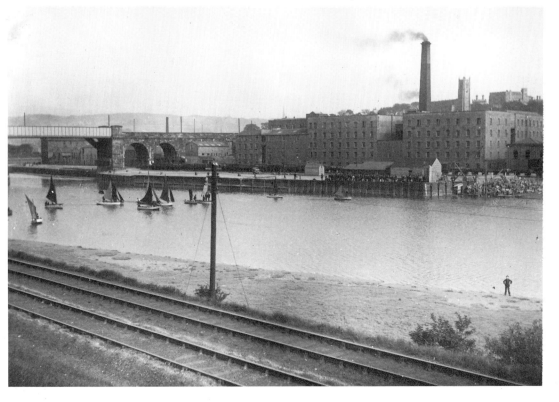

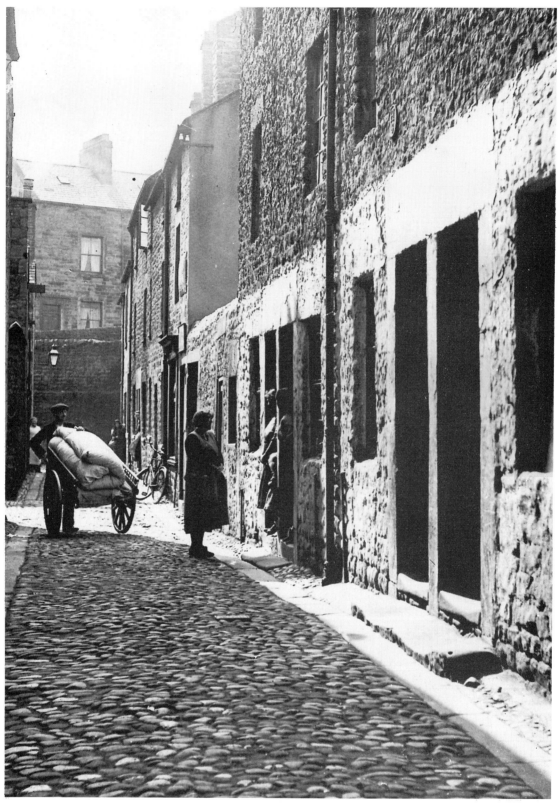

122.   River Street, off St George's Quay. This was an area of cheap housing and attracted some of the poorer families. It was often subject to flooding, and still is on occasion. Many of the smaller houses have now gone and warehouses, built in the 18th century to handle the cargoes from the West Indies, have been turned into flats.

Transport

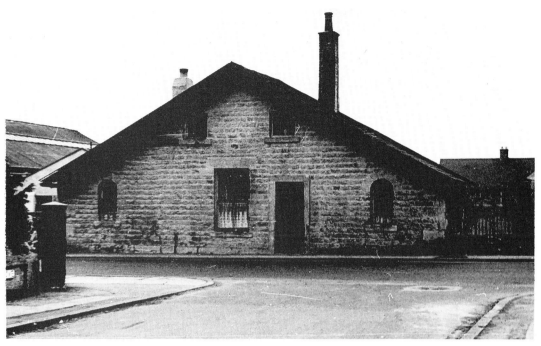

123. Toll Bar Cottage at Scotforth, photographed in February 1952. The cottage has long since been demolished and Toll Bar Garage now stands on the site. The design of the cottage is similar to that of the one which survives just to the north of Garstang. It is probably a standard type for the Garstang and Heron Syke Turnpike of 1750.

124. The *King's Arms Hotel*'s private horse bus, used for fetching visitors from the railway stations.

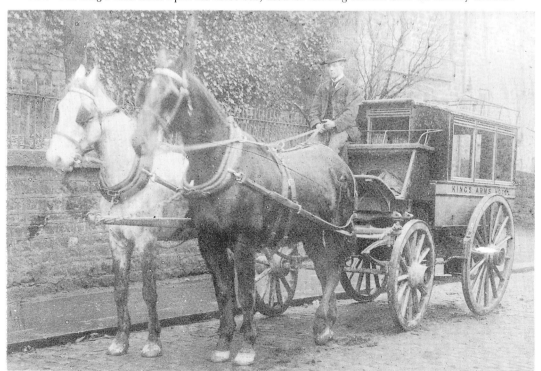

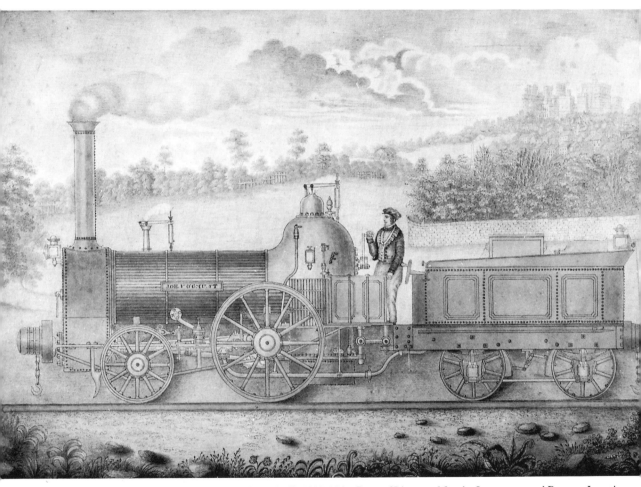

125. A drawing of the locomotive *John O'Gaunt*, built 1839-40 by Bury of Liverpool for the Lancaster and Preston Junction Railway. *John O'Gaunt* was one of six locomotives bought for the opening of the new railway line and was one of those sold in 1849 when the company ceased to operate the line. This drawing may possibly have been produced for the sale of the locomotive.

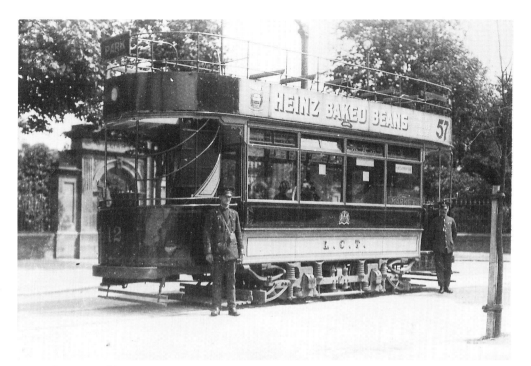

126. Lancaster City tram car no. 12 at Williamson Park gates. Driver Williams is on the right. The tram cars ran from 1903 to 1930, but were never a great success because Lancaster was too small and hilly.

127. A 'coffin car' at Scotforth. Coffin cars were single-deck trams, their shape giving rise to their macabre name. They were introduced in 1920.

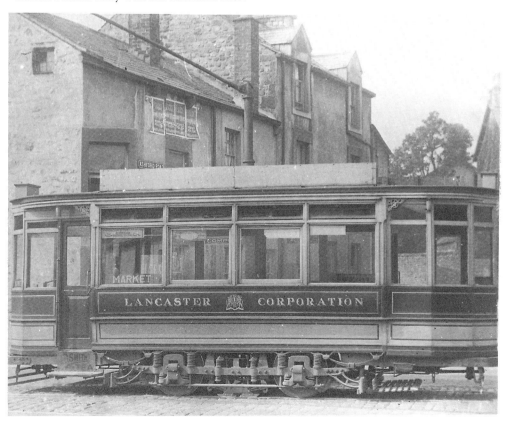

Fire Brigade

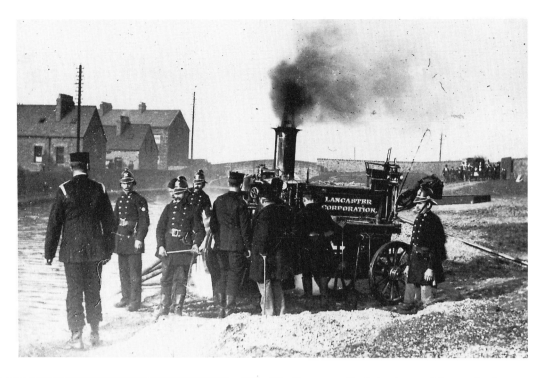

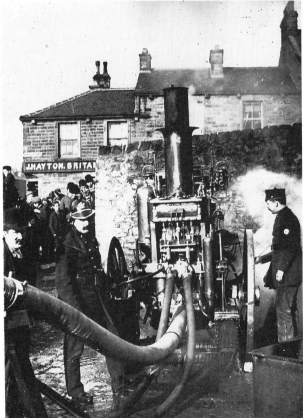

128. The Lancaster fire brigade exercising at the dry dock on the Lancaster Canal, probably in the 1890s. The dry dock was built for the repair of canal barges. Chief Constable Harris is supervising operations.

129. Lancaster fire brigade in action in Ullswater Road on the Freehold in the 1890s. Their steam-operated pump was made by Shand Mason & Co. of London.

Health Care

130. Gardyner's Chantry in St Mary's Gate. The chantry was founded in 1485 by John Gardyner. The almshouses, which formed part of the chantry, were rebuilt in 1792 in the form seen here. The four almshouses have now been demolished, and all that is left of them is the plaque from the front which is set into the wall of a building in the gardens of the Old Vicarage.

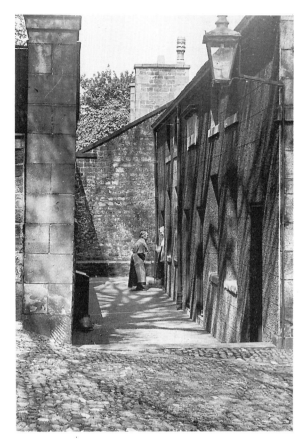

131. Gillison's Hospital, almshouses for women which stood until 1960 in Common Garden Street. The almshouses were demolished in that year and were rebuilt in Lindow Square. They were founded in 1790 under the will of the late Mrs. Ann Gillison and consisted originally of eight 'very neat houses built round a quadrangle court for eight unmarried women'.

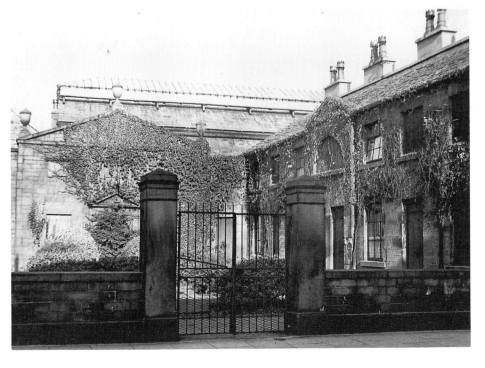

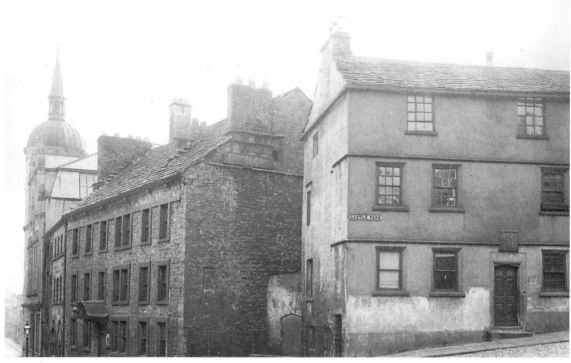

132. Castle Park, showing the houses demolished in 1906 to make way for the extension to the Storey Institute. Houses on this corner originally belonged to merchant families, such as the Rawlinsons. The building to the right was used as the Dispensary from 1781 until 1785. This was supported by subscriptions and provided basic health care for the poor. Up to 1,400 patients were treated here in an average year.

133. A small neat building on Castle Hill which was completed in 1785 and served as the Dispensary until 1833. Over the door was originally set a relief of the Good Samaritan, now at the Royal Lancaster Infirmary.

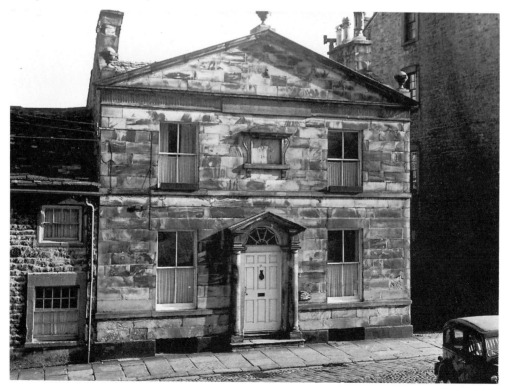

134. The coade stone plaque showing the Good Samaritan, now over the door to the Royal Lancaster Infirmary. It has been moved to successive buildings as the Dispensary has required more room, but probably dates from the 1780s.

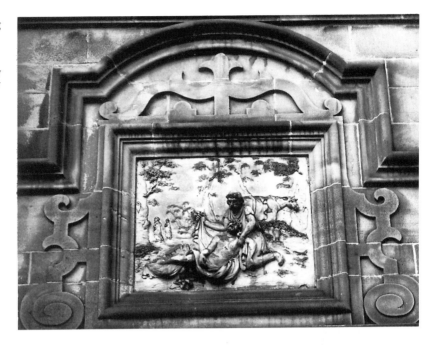

135. Thurnham Street, showing the town house of Lord Viscount Fauconberg and the Dispensary. This Dispensary replaced the building on Castle Hill in 1833. The tall building further down the street to the right is the birthplace of Sir Richard Owen, coiner of the word 'dinosaur'. The low building on the left has been replaced by the *Royal Hotel*.

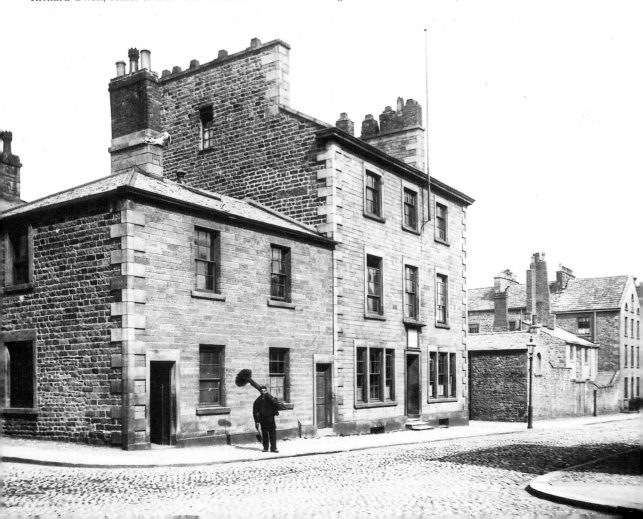

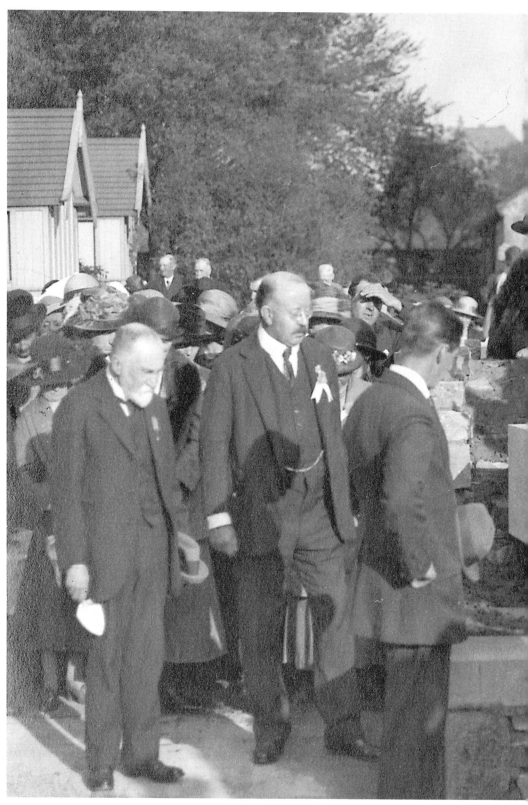

136 Laying the foundation stone of the Royal Lancaster Infirmary. The building was officially opened in 1896 by the Duke and Duchess of York. The original building is now surrounded by a vast complex of hospital buildings, as Lancaster is an important centre for health care.

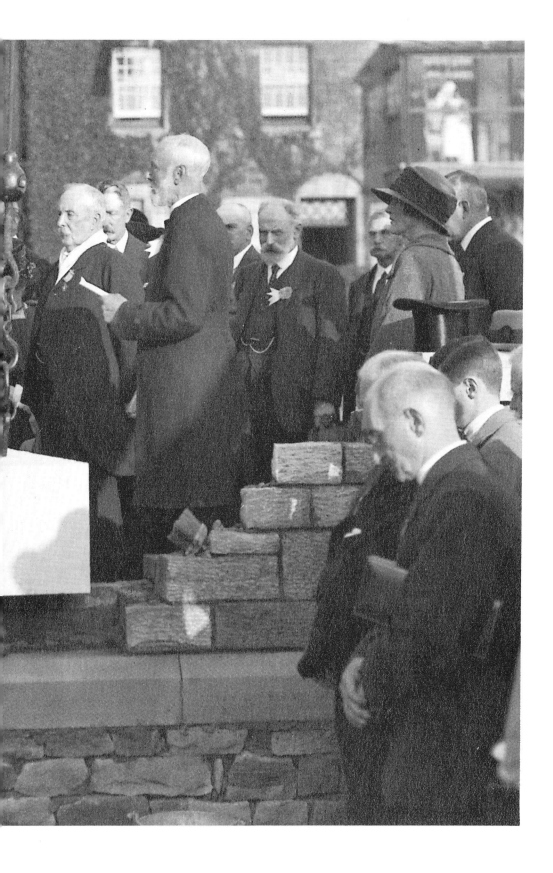

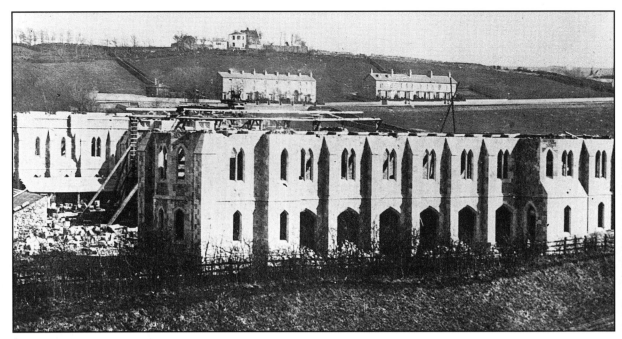

137. Ripley Hospital under construction, some time between 1856 and 1864. The houses in the background are in Bowerham Road and South Road. This is an exceptionally interesting photograph because of its early date.

138. Ripley Hospital, built by J. Cunningham at the expense of Mrs. Julia Ripley. Parts of the building complex are now used as Ripley St Thomas School, but it was originally an orphanage.

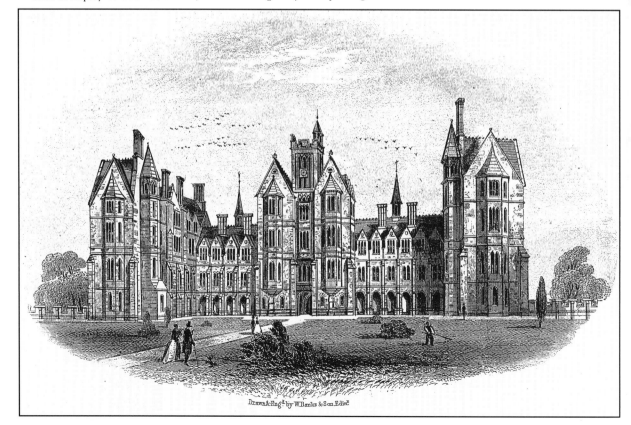

Drawn & Engd by W. Banks & Son. Edinr

Sports and Pastimes

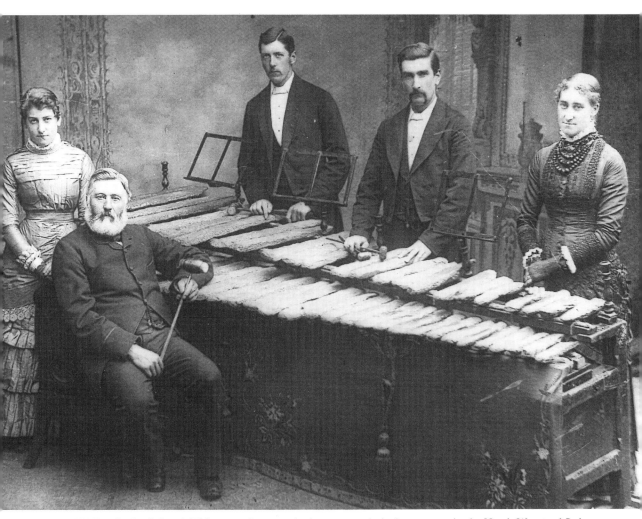

139. The Till Family Rock Band. This type of stone xylophone was relatively common in the North West and Lake District, and several sets of tuned stones have survived. The stones themselves were selected from particular limestone outcrops, such as Kendal Fell, where the stones were found to have a distinct musical tone which could be tuned. They were played by several players, each taking care of an octave or so. The Till Family Rock Band toured America and Europe and had several rivals, including Richardson's Original Rock Band.

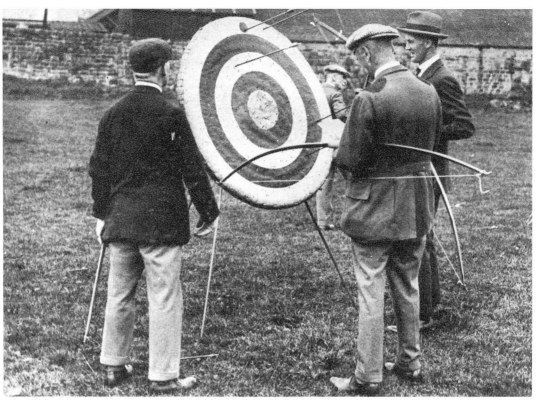

140. The John O'Gaunt Bowmen, seen here on their field day in 1930, totting up the scores.

141. An unposed photograph on the same day, looking down the range. The John O'Gaunt Bowmen are one of Lancaster's oldest sporting clubs, originating in 1788. They originally practised in Springfield Park, moving in the 1850s to a field off Meeting House Lane.

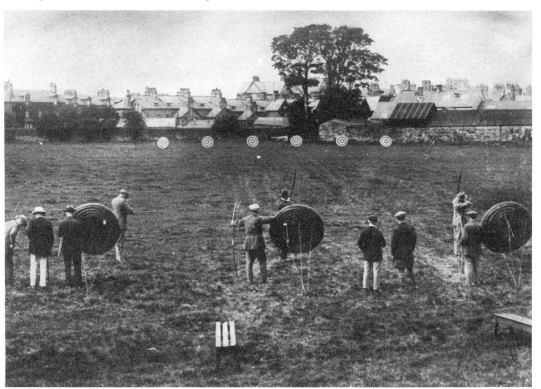

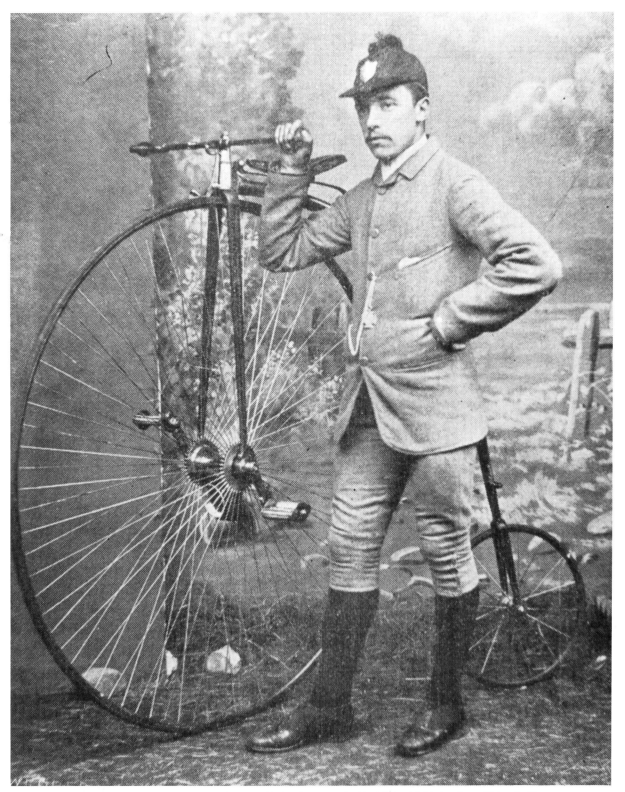

142. S. Dawson, captain of the Lancaster Cycling Club, photographed in 1880 with his 'ordinary' bicycle. Dawson wrote a most illuminating account of the early days of cycling, which appeared under the title of *Incidents in the Course of a Long Cycling Career*. He was captain for 19 years and records that the members of the cycling club had caps trimmed with silver lace, with silver badges, while the captain had gold lace and gold badges.

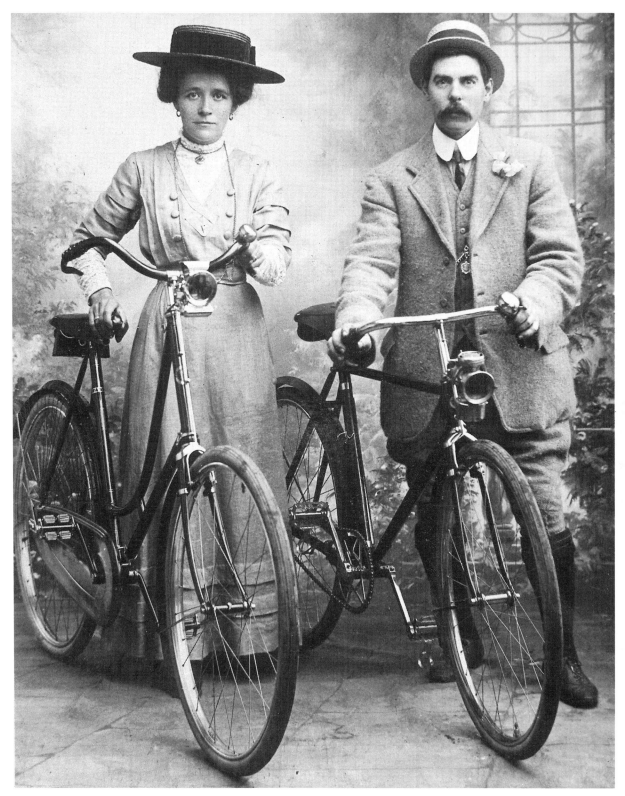

143. William and Jenny Clarkson, of the Williamson Park Cycling Club, 1910-12. The Park Cycling Club was very popular in the Edwardian period and many married couples were members. William Clarkson worked at Storeys and lived on the Freehold. His bicycle had a bamboo wheel, back pedal brake and three-speed hub gearing. William was killed in an explosion in the 1950s.

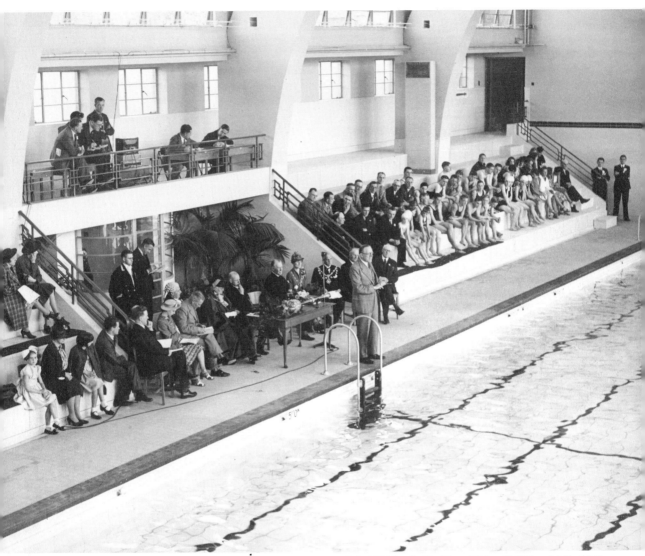

144. The opening of the public swimming baths at Kingsway on 1 July 1939 by the Rt. Hon. Walter E. Elliott M.C., M.P., Minister of Health. The Kingsway baths were the first swimming baths in Lancaster, and the complex, providing room for a variety of other sporting activities, is now known as the Kingsway Centre.

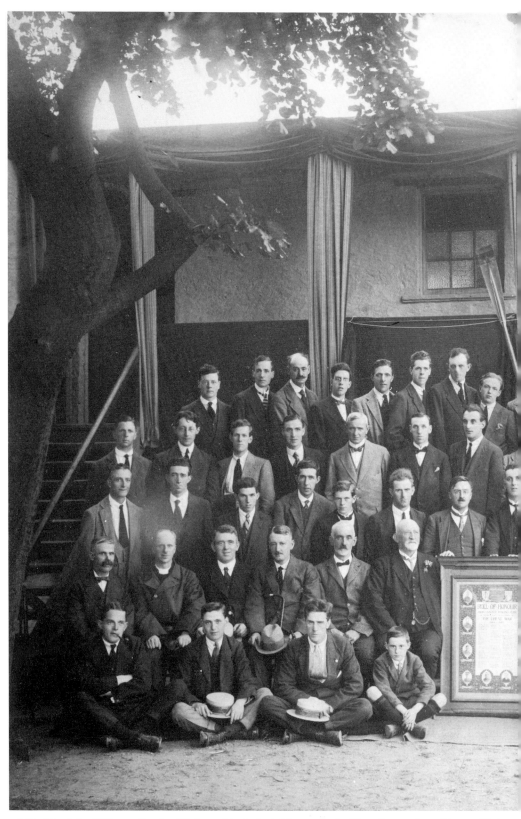

145. The John O'Gaunt Rowing Club outside their clubhouse on the River Lune, above Skerton Weirs, in the 1920s. Although not the oldest of Lancaster's rowing clubs, the John O'Gaunt has proved to be the longest lived. It was founded in 1867. The club used the fine stretch of the Lune leading through the aqueduct, known as Halton Water.

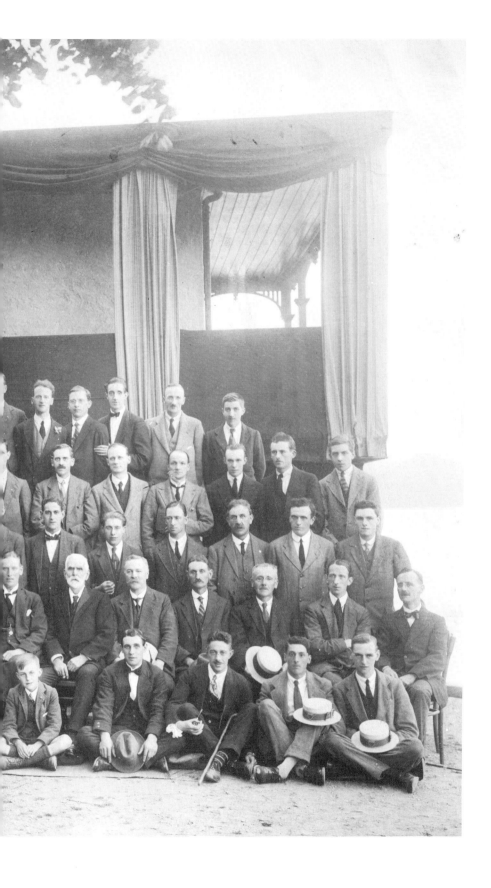

Heysham

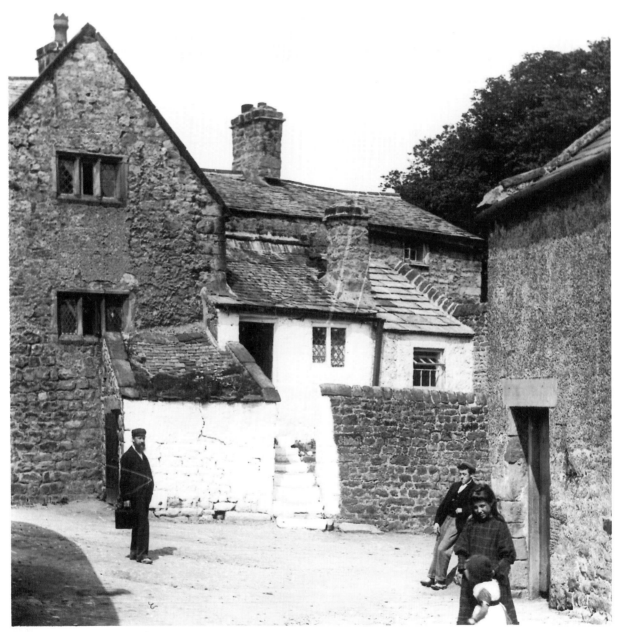

146.   The Old Rectory at Heysham, otherwise known as Greese House (from the Anglo-Saxon for 'steps'), built in 1680. Heysham village has long been a magnet for tourists, and has managed very largely to avoid the urbanising influence of Morecambe, its immediate neighbour to the north. However, the old village is now just a picturesque centre of a large suburban area.

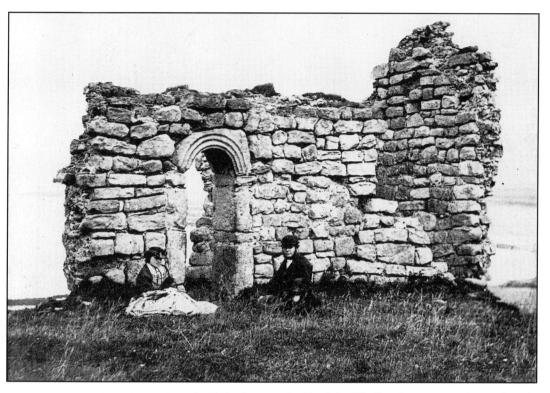

147. St Patrick's Chapel, Heysham, in 1861, photographed by J. L. Whalley. Some restoration work took place in 1903, but otherwise the building is little changed today.

148. The atmospheric ruin of St Patrick's Chapel. Although the connection with St Patrick cannot be substantiated, this is clearly a very important site of considerable antiquity. On this headland are the only two Anglo-Saxon churches in Lancashire. St Peter's, the parish church, lies lower down, while on the rocky heights above stands St Patrick's Chapel, of which only three walls survive. Excavation here in 1977 and 1978 showed that the present ruin belongs to a rebuilt chapel and its origins are even earlier. The chapel had painted wall plaster and there were a number of rock-cut graves, many of which can be seen today. Outside the door in this photograph a hollow containing many burials was excavated, in which was found a Viking bone comb. Both church and chapel date from between the seventh and ninth centuries.

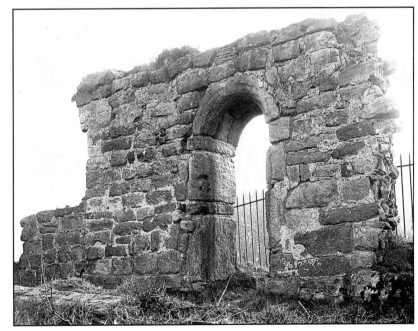

Morecambe

149.   Morecambe, from the entrance to the stone jetty. This view, one of a series published in a coloured booklet, probably in the early 1870s, shows the original station at the end of the pier, built in 1848, with its lighthouse and attendant sheds. Considerable, and perhaps exaggerated, shipping activity is taking place in the bay. The jetty served as a ferry terminal for boats to Fleetwood, the Isle of Man, Ireland and Scotland. The railway was one of the principal reasons for Morecambe's meteoric growth in the second half of the 19th century.

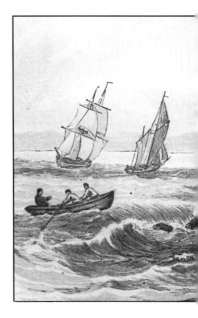

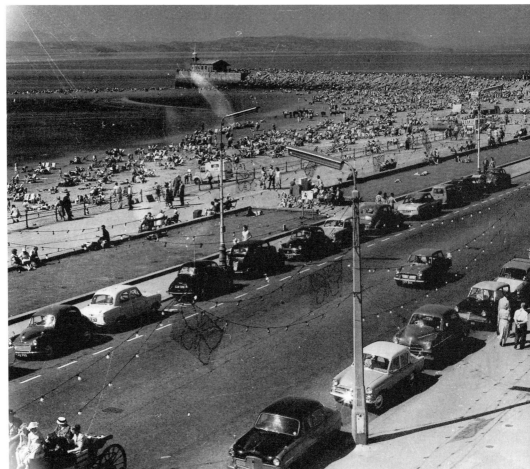

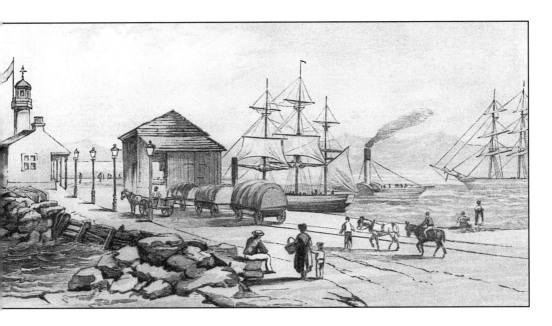

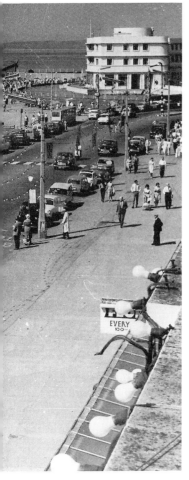

150. A busy holiday time in Morecambe, *c*.1960. This was the peak period for seaside resorts, when post-war affluence began to be felt, and before package tours to foreign, and particularly Spanish, resorts developed. To the left can be seen one of the horse-drawn landaus, which used to ply for trade along the promenade. To the right of the picture is the *Midland Hotel* of 1932-3, by Oliver Hill, and stretching away from it to the sea is the stone jetty, the original railway pier built in 1848 as a ferry terminal.

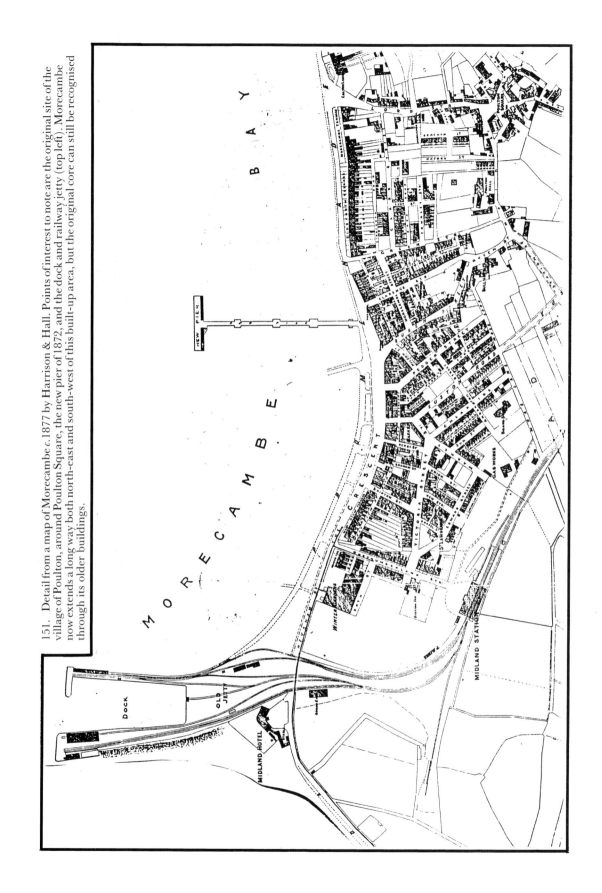

151. Detail from a map of Morecambe c.1877 by Harrison & Hall. Points of interest to note are the original site of the village of Poulton, around Poulton Square, the new pier of 1872, and the dock and railway jetty (top left). Morecambe now extends a long way both north-east and south-west of this built-up area, but the original core can still be recognised through its older buildings.

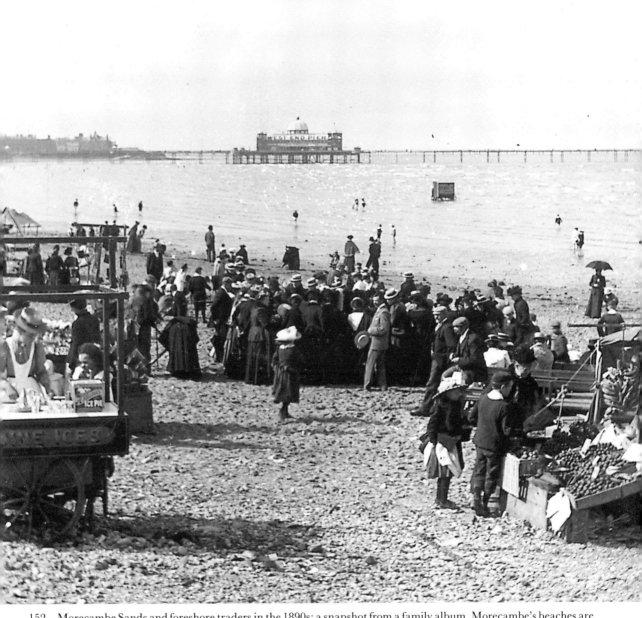

152. Morecambe Sands and foreshore traders in the 1890s: a snapshot from a family album. Morecambe's beaches are subject to a cycle of erosion and deposition which depends on the movement of the deep river channels out in the bay. At present works are in progress to break the force of storm surges and encourage the deposition of sand.

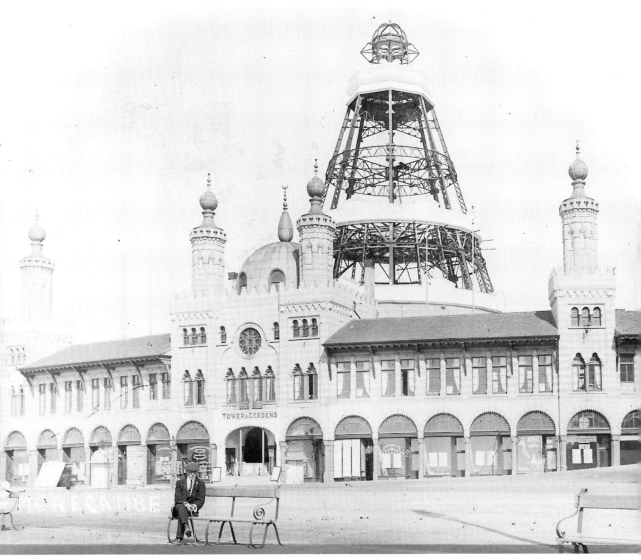

153. Morecambe Tower and gardens, 1910. Blackpool was not alone in having a tower! A grandiose scheme for a 232-ft. tower in Morecambe was launched in 1898 but the project was never completed. The site is now marked by the Granada building close to Morecambe Town Hall.

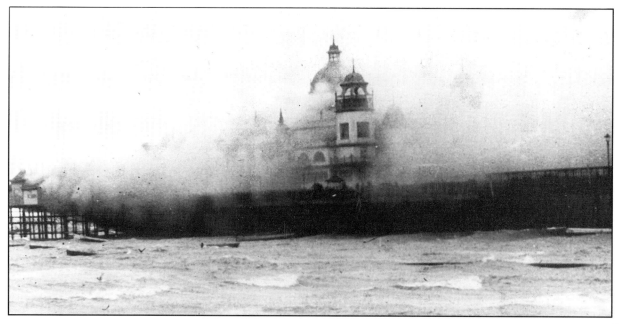

154. Morecambe Pier on fire in 1933: a sad end to a fine structure which formed the seaward end of the Central Pier. In 1988 another fire severely damaged its successor.

155. The West End Pier, built in 1896, a tangled ruin after the storm of November 1977. The shallow waters of Morecambe Bay are prone to sudden storm surges. All traces of the pier have now gone.

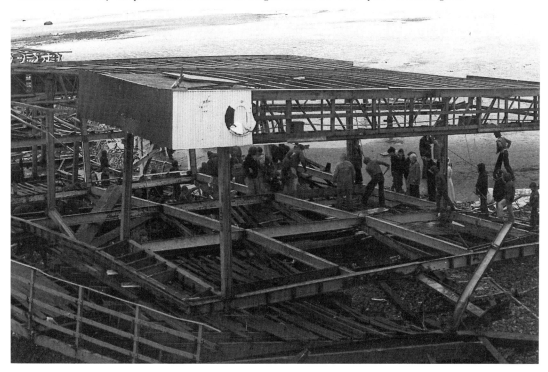

Skerton

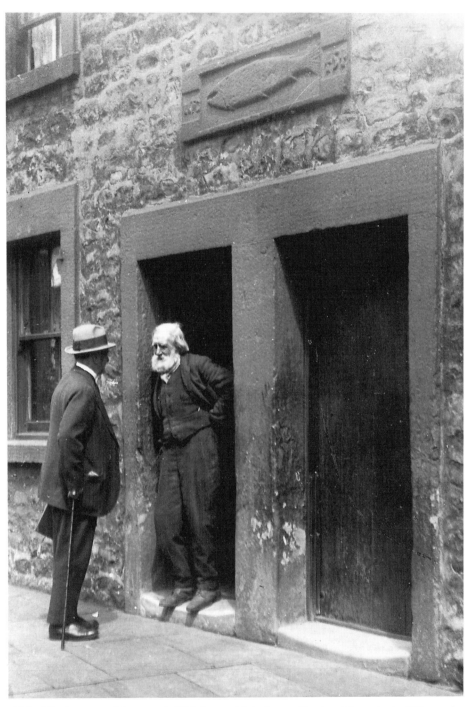

156.   The doorway of the water bailiff's house, Main Street, Skerton. The water bailiff served the Beaumont fishery, originally established by Furness Abbey in the 12th century. It was a very valuable possession, because of the richness of the salmon fishing in the River Lune. The lintel stone, carved with a salmon and the date 1651, can now be seen at Lancaster Maritime Museum.

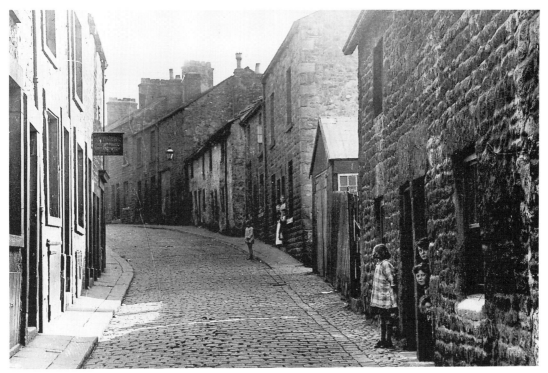

157. Main Street, Skerton. Skerton is the suburb of Lancaster lying north of the river. This part was altered out of all recognition around 1960 during major replanning of the suburb. At that time much of its village character was lost.

158. Captain's Row, 1927. An atmospheric picture, showing delivery of barrels by dray. Captain's Row lay north-west of the northern end of Skerton Bridge.

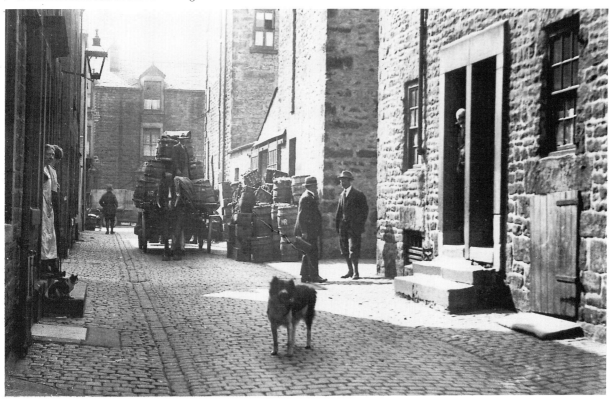

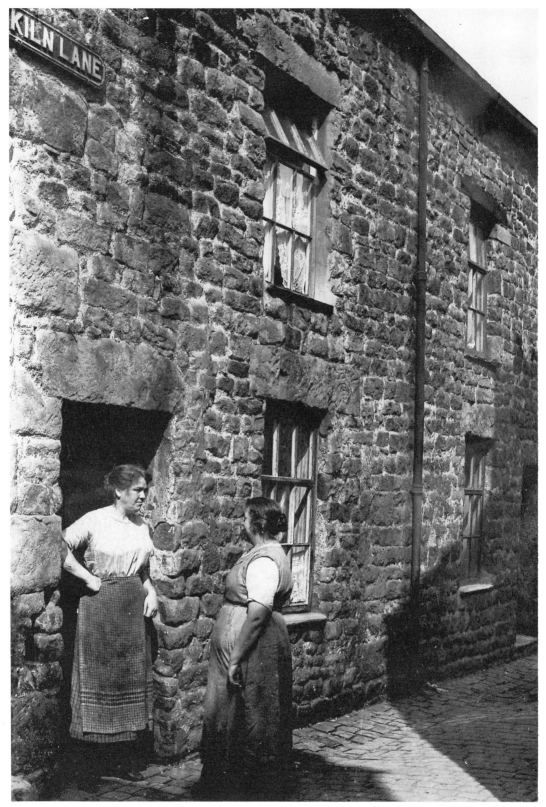

159. Kiln Lane in Skerton. These houses were demolished in 1960 during redevelopment. Their rugged stone construction was typical of the area. Kiln Lane was probably named from Robert Aldren's malt-kiln, which stood here in the early 19th century.

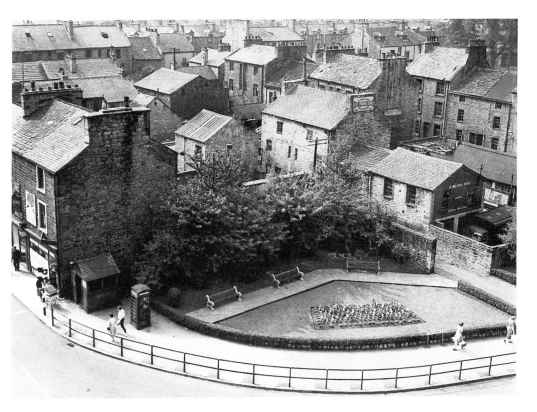

160. The junction of Owen Road and Morecambe Road from the tower of Skerton Methodist church. In the background are Kiln Lane and Captain's Row, but since this photograph was taken in the 1950s the whole area has been totally changed and most of the buildings demolished.

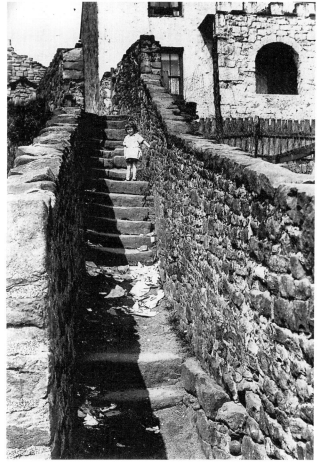

161. Drinkwater Steps, Skerton. These steps linked Main Street with the Ramparts, the area next to the river, and came out by the *Blue Anchor*.

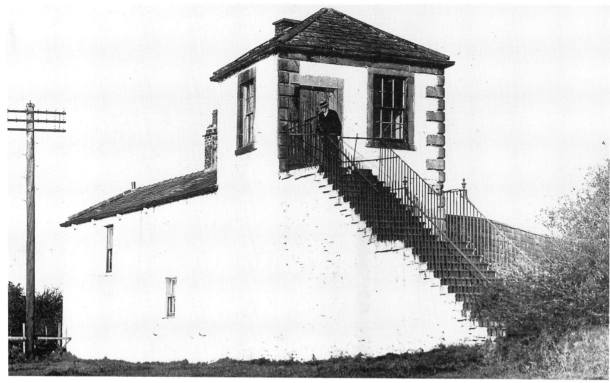

162. Mount Pleasant, Skerton: a little tower-like building which stood opposite the end of Vale Road on the present A6. The man on the steps in this 1920s' photograph is Jack Manley.

163. Skerton tan yards in the snow in 1894. There were two tan yards at Skerton, with traditional timber slatted buildings and tanning pits. Both have now disappeared.

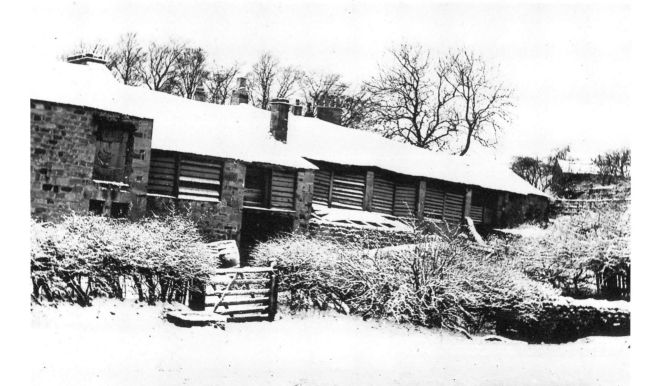

Scotforth

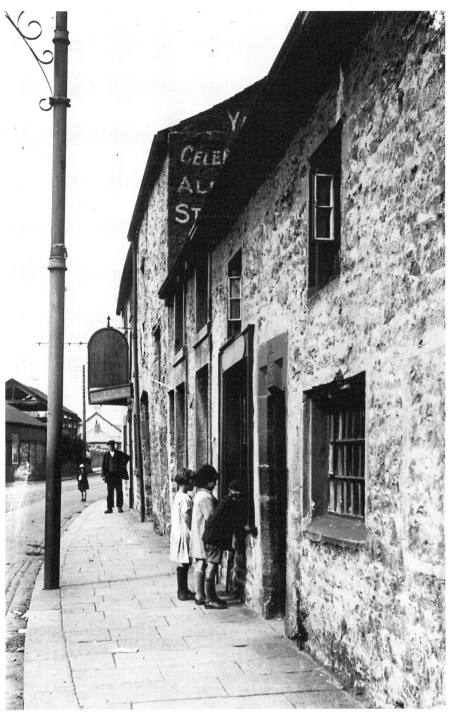

164. The *Bowling Green Hotel* at Scotforth, *c.*1927-30. A typical dated lintel reading B/IS 1676 can be seen towards the middle of the picture.

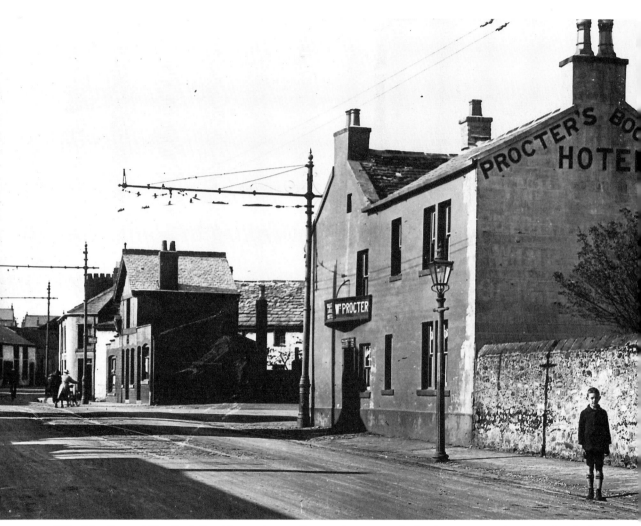

165. The *Boot and Shoe Hotel*. Outside are the tramlines and tram standards; the trams terminated at Scotforth.

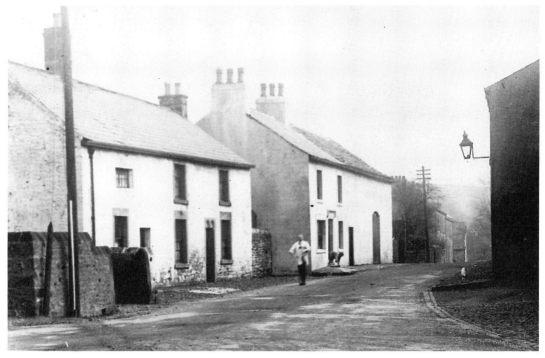

166. Hala Road, Scotforth. Scotforth was for a long time a village, separate from Lancaster. Tentacles of urban growth gradually united the two, but Scotforth still retains some of its village character. Hala Road still exists but leads now to a large post-war housing estate.

167. The site of Scotforth Pottery. The Pottery was set up in the 1840s, and for some years was run by potters of the Bateson family from Burton in Lonsdale. The kiln probably lay to the right of the cottages where the rather curious curved wall can be seen. The whole scene has been transformed since this photograph was taken.

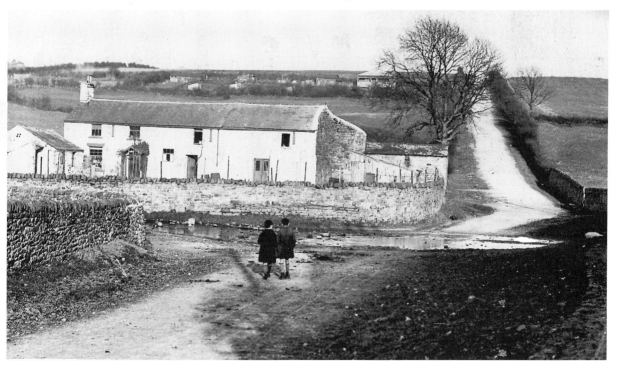

The Lune Valley

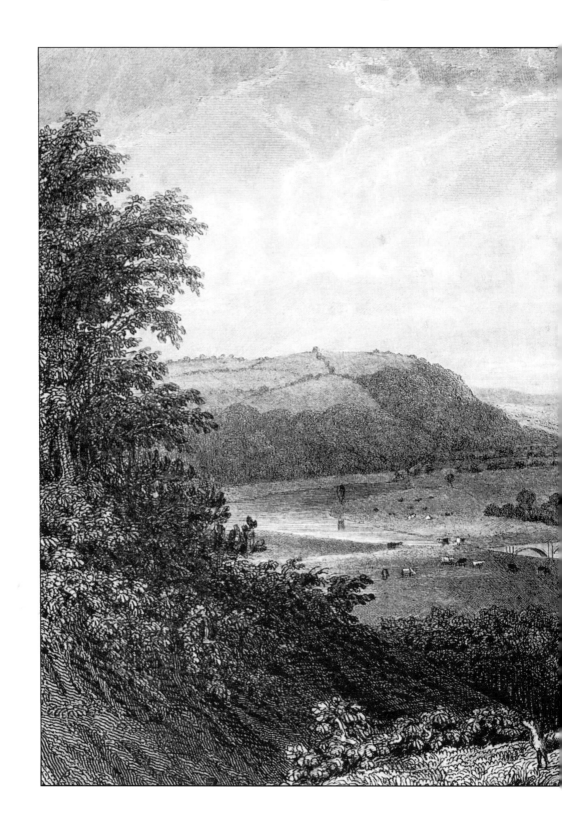

168. The Vale of Lonsdale, from an engraving after J. Henderson. This view, a popular one with 18th- and 19th-century travellers, opened out to the north-east from a point three miles from Lancaster, near the village of Caton. The road has now changed, but the beauties of the Lune Valley continue to delight travellers today.

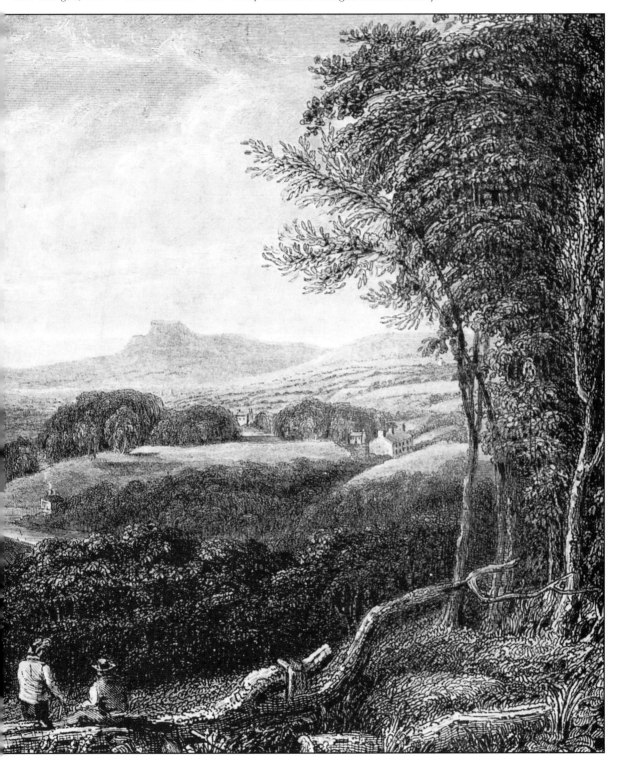

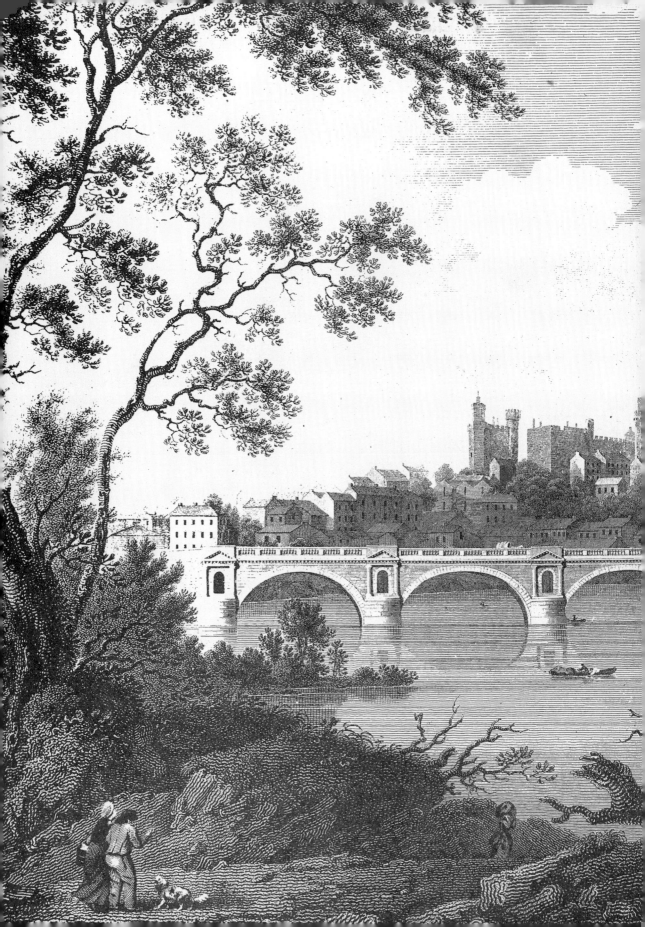